WHY
CAESAREAN
MATTERS

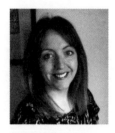

About the author

Clare Goggin was inspired to write this book following her own caesarean births. She was curious about whether caesarean birth experiences could be improved, so she created a space on social media where healthcare professionals and women could explore this together.

She has been invited to speak at the Positive Birth Movement's 'Be the Change' conference, as well as to local obstetricians and midwives, and has written about caesarean birth for *Juno* magazine and the *British Journal of Midwifery*.

She also draws on her extensive experiences of working to improve maternal heath in the NHS and third sector prior to having children, including supporting the implementation of local and national improvement programmes, such as Maternity Matters.

Clare Goggin can be contacted via Twitter at @msclaregoggin

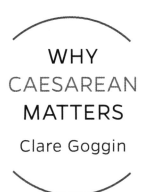

WHY
CAESAREAN
MATTERS

Clare Goggin

Why Caesarean Matters (Pinter & Martin Why It Matters 12)

First published by Pinter & Martin Ltd 2018

ISBN 978-1-78066-540-5

Also available as an ebook

Pinter & Martin Why It Matters ISSN 2056-8657
Series editor: Susan Last
Index: Helen Bilton
Cover Design: Blok Graphic, London
Cover illustration: Sam Kalda

British Library Cataloguing-in-Publication Data

A catalogue record for this book is available from the British Library.

Set in Minion

Printed and bound in the EU by Hussar

This book has been printed on paper that is sourced and harvested from sustainable forests and is FSC accredited.

Pinter & Martin Ltd
6 Effra Parade
London SW2 1PS
pinterandmartin.com

Contents

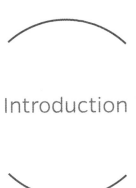

Introduction

As you might expect of a woman-centred book about caesarean birth, this book is both personal and political.

I offer you my personal perspective – a perspective that has grown out of my own caesarean birth experiences, and through listening to the experiences of hundreds of other women. I write carefully and humbly, drawing heavily on the existing evidence base surrounding birth, yet I also know that I cannot convey the full complexity of the caesarean birth experience in this short book.

Rather, this book is an invitation.

My hope is that the words I write here will draw out *your* words, whether you are currently pregnant; are someone who has birthed by caesarean; or are working in maternity care. Or, indeed, all three.

In hoping to draw out your words, this book is also political. I agree with Rebecca Solnit when she wrote: '*a valued person lives in a society in which her story has a place*'.[1] Sharing our birth stories is political because a society (and a health system) that values the birth stories of women, values women.

Birth is something that everyone has a stake in, both as individuals (because we all owe our lives to pregnancy and birth) and as citizens (via our taxes). Yet we (as a society) rarely imagine birth experiences through the eyes of the woman at the centre.

As pregnant women (and throughout motherhood), we are subject to the 'gaze' of others. Our decisions are analysed, and sometimes praised, but all too often found wanting. This is true for all of us, whether we birth vaginally or via caesarean. This 'gaze' can feel incredibly intense for those of us making decisions about (or recovering from) caesarean birth. We are acutely aware that caesarean birth is often considered to be 'birth gone wrong'.

In truth, though, caesarean birth is neither right nor wrong. It is paradoxical. Caesarean birth can be both beneficial and detrimental. Those who choose caesarean birth can struggle to feel heard, while those who seek to avoid a caesarean often feel the same. Caesarean birth is endlessly debated and scrutinised, yet many mothers who give birth by caesarean feel unable to talk about their experiences – be they positive or negative.

Too often caesarean birth is presented as both forbidden and compulsory. It need not be. There is another way to frame caesarean birth, a way that honours *you*, the woman at the centre of birth. This book has been written to help you find it.

Who is this book for?

Although this book is written for anyone with an interest in compassionate, woman-centred caesarean birth, I have had two groups at the forefront of my mind.

The first group is *pregnant women*. You are pregnant, possibly for the first time, and it's both exciting and daunting. You are making decisions about your birth and navigating the wealth of research and opinion that's available. Caesarean birth might be a distant possibility. Or you may be reading this because you are planning a caesarean birth or weighing up a recommendation from your caregivers. I hope you enjoy the book and that it helps you feel prepared to have a positive birth experience,[2] regardless of its clinical outcome.

The second group is *those who have birthed by caesarean*. We are not all the same, we women who birth by caesarean. Each of us will have our own stories and I hope that there will be something in this book for all of you. You may have given birth by caesarean yesterday, or it may have been many years ago. It may have been hoped for, planned for or completely unexpected. It may have been a straightforward procedure or it may have been complex. You may be planning further pregnancies or you might not. The variations are truly endless.

We have different world-views too. Some of us were (and might still be) passionate about 'natural' or 'normal' birth, while others may be equally passionate about the value of medical assistance. In writing this book, I have really tried to think about caesarean birth from as many angles as possible and to take on board the diversity of experiences women have.

Why have I included self-care questions?

I know from personal experience how easy it is to become overwhelmed with feelings of fear, confusion and disconnection when exploring this topic. There are so many opinions that are so fiercely held, that we can feel completely at sea. As Glosswitch wrote in the *New Statesman*: *'pity the laboring woman, caught in the middle of this! Who can she trust?'*

Understanding caesarean birth requires both a search for evidence and for meaning. And so, I try to open up the debates and controversies; encourage you to have meaningful discussions with your caregivers; and also to encourage you to create space for reflection and forming your own judgments about what is important to you.

How to use the self-care questions

- There is no single way to use them. You could sit in meditation, you could go for a walk in nature, you could ponder them while washing up or chat them through with a friend.
- A notebook and pen may be helpful, either to help you remember any questions you have for your caregiver, or to help you make sense of your thoughts.
- These questions can be used alongside other mindfulness approaches (birth-focused or otherwise); they are simply intended to draw out a caesarean-specific perspective.
- The questions may not work for everyone. If you are struggling, please do talk to your midwife, health visitor or GP to access specialist support to work through your experiences in a way that feels safe for you.

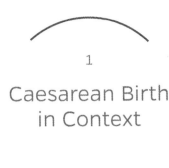

1

Caesarean Birth
in Context

Caesarean birth can be difficult to talk about. There is a pervasive idea that women are engaged in 'birth wars', in which our personal preferences and decisions about our births become overly politicised and place us in conflict with each other. Many women I speak to feel exhausted by the way that the debate surrounding caesarean birth is framed. We simply want the best possible birth for ourselves and our babies, in light of our individual circumstances.

Yet there are 'political' questions to explore surrounding birth – though I wish they could be less focused on 'what should she do?' and more focused on 'how can we support her?' Birth is political because it involves more than one person. The overwhelming majority of women seek out the support of others during birth[1] (whether from a partner, doula, midwife and/or obstetric team). How do we define the roles of each of these actors in birth? How do they relate to each other? How do they relate to the mother at the centre of birth? How do we understand the relationship between the mother and her baby (or babies)? These are all questions that challenge us to consider the power dynamics in modern birth.

As Vanessa Olorenshaw perceptively noted in her must-read book *Liberating Motherhood*: '*at times, we can feel that we are on the sidelines, listening to political discussion about our lives and shaking our heads because it doesn't speak for us.*' [2]

This is exactly how I feel when I hear many discussions about caesarean birth. I often find myself wincing, as my own experience of caesarean birth is so much more complex than is often presented. We have to speak for ourselves. We don't all have to agree or value the same things. The power I am seeking is simply my own power, and that's all I would wish for you too. So let's start by looking at the big questions in the current debate surrounding caesarean birth. Why are caesarean birth rates rising? What is caesarean birth like in other parts of the world? Then we will start to consider how these debates are shifting towards a much more woman-centred model of care, asking: How can I make informed choices? How can I have a voice in my care?

Self-care questions
- How does the debate surrounding caesarean birth make me feel?
- What steps can I take to support myself emotionally as I think about caesarean birth?
- How open am I to changing my mind about caesarean birth?
- How do I feel about the possibility of having a voice in (or about) my birth?

Why are caesarean birth rates increasing?

Over the past 65 years, birth has changed in a fundamental way: caesarean birth is now commonplace, with more than 174,000 caesarean births in 2016/17 in England alone.[3] That's the equivalent to almost 20 births every hour! In the 1950s, just

3% of births were via caesarean[4] and in 2018 this had risen to over a quarter.[5]

This dramatic shift has attracted a lot of attention from healthcare professionals, government policymakers and grassroots campaigners, all of whom are asking: 'Why are caesarean birth rates rising?'

Some argue that rising caesarean rates are underpinned by factors relating to the mother: older mothers; more 'high-risk' mothers;[6] more women affected by obesity; the impact of repeat caesareans; and consumer choice. Others disagree, as Rebecca Schiller writes:

> With predictable regularity, every time the caesarean rate is mentioned, women are blamed... But for most women, keen to have as uncomplicated a birth as possible, current practice often leads to a caesarean that they may not have needed yet will probably be reported as a failure within their bodies rather than the system.[7]

Reframing the caesarean birth rate debate

In all my discussions with policymakers, healthcare professionals, campaigners and mothers alike, I have observed a conundrum at the centre of caesarean birth discussions: few stakeholders deny that caesarean birth can save lives, but many stakeholders disagree about how and when this happens.

I find myself reflecting that we often talk about caesarean birth as if it is *the problem*. It isn't. Not even a little bit. It is *a solution*. What is it a solution to? In my opinion, it is a solution to two challenges:

- Risks to life in pregnancy and birth; and
- Uncertainty in pregnancy and birth.

Risks to life of mother and baby
Let's start with understanding the relationship between caesarean and risks to life during pregnancy and birth. The table below summarises what we know about the relationship between caesarean rates and risks to life for mother and baby (when looking at large populations), using the World Health Organization's (WHO) 2015 Statement of Caesarean Section Rates.[8]

Caesarean birth rate	Impact on risks to life for mother and baby
<10%	Increasing caesarean rates associated with less risk to life for mother and baby.
10 to 30%	No difference in risk to life for mother and baby (not worse, but also not better). A study (published later in 2015 than the WHO statement) suggested that rates of up to 19% were associated with lower maternal and neonatal mortality rates based on all 194 WHO member states.[9]
> 30%	We don't know enough to say.

Note: The WHO analysis also notes that we do not fully understand the relationship between caesarean birth rates and other non-mortality related outcomes (such as the on-going impact on physical, developmental and/or emotional health outcomes).

We can look at the information above in at least two ways. Firstly, we can ask: why do more than a quarter of women give birth by caesarean, when there is limited evidence that such a high rate is beneficial? Secondly, why is there such a huge debate about caesarean birth rates when there is so little robust evidence that it is harmful?

It's quite the conundrum. It seems as though our debates surrounding caesarean have often got stuck here. However, we also need to remember that we don't make decisions about caesarean birth at a population level. These decisions are made one by one, leading me to a far more interesting question: How do caregivers and pregnant women work together to make decisions during pregnancy and birth?

Uncertainty in pregnancy and birth

There is a contradiction at the heart of decision-making in birth.

On the one hand, women's bodies are incredibly effective at birthing healthy babies. Adverse outcomes for babies are uncommon[10] and the *Lancet* recently noted that a '*man is much more likely to die while his partner is pregnant than she is.*'[11] Indeed, if we look at rates of neonatal and maternal mortality for women living in 'fragile and conflict-affected situations' (where outcomes for maternal health are among the worst in the world and we might not expect widespread caesarean access), we might be surprised that they are some way off 10-15% (let alone 27%).[12]

On the other hand, it is equally clear that devastating outcomes can occur, and that most of these outcomes appear to be preventable. The RCOG Each Baby Counts project seeks to reduce the number of babies that die or are left severely disabled, due to events that occur in birth. Their 2015 report found that different care may have impacted the outcome in 76% of the cases that they reviewed.[13]

Our questions as pregnant women (for example: 'Is a caesarean medically necessary?') are not always clear cut to answer. Sure, there are some circumstances that are rarely contested: for example, if a woman has placenta praevia,[14] but in others, such as a woman birthing a breech baby, when a baby has an unusual heart rate or in the management of a long labour, there is much more disagreement. Indeed, recent analysis of US and UK Obstetrics and Gynaecology guidelines reveals that only a minority of recommendations are based on high-quality, consistent evidence.[15]

This highlights to me that decisions about caesarean birth are not always an exact science, and can often be made as a way of 'hedging our bets' against a possibly much worse outcome.[16] Just like we sometimes give prophylactic antibiotics to prevent an infection, sometimes we recommend (as caregivers) or choose (as pregnant women) a caesarean to prevent a possible adverse outcome.

As Florence Wilcock (consultant obstetrician and co-founder of the #matexp movement to improve birth) describes:

My job is to master the art of being there only at the critical time, to run in and save the day, keep calm whilst doing so and to never get that judgement wrong. An impossible balance of risk vs choice, art vs science, clinical outcome vs maternal experience.[17]

The fact that we make risk-averse choices about pregnancy and childbirth, and that this may lead us to intervene 'just in case', is not inherently good or bad. The challenge begins when we ask: Whose decision is it?

While the legal position is clear that the final decision lies in our hands (see p22), as pregnant women, the reality is that we rely on our caregivers to inform and support our decisions. And what do our caregivers rely upon? Obstetrician Dr Amali Lokugamage notes that:

[in the western world at least] contemporary healthcare is now being driven by a technocratic model where complex health, social, political and economic elements are protocolised, guided by risk, cost and fear, at the expense of personalised care.[18]

Moreover, I have heard many women talk about feeling that the decisions about their birth are made by healthcare professionals *for them*, rather than *with them*.[19]

This is what I hope to challenge, and I know many other campaigners, policy-makers and healthcare professionals do too. This is where I believe we will achieve some of the most positive change in maternity care and the best possible outcomes for women and their babies.

What do we lose in the politics of percentages?

If we focus only on percentage rates when we discuss caesarean birth, we can become unable to see the diverse stories of women who birth by caesarean. In particular, we run the risk of:

Unintended consequences

All government policy decisions and priorities have unintended consequences (after all, humans and the institutions we create are incredibly complex). Thankfully, key stakeholders from the World Health Organization to the Department of Health have recognised the potential for negative unintended consequences if we were to set a target caesarean birth rate.

Not only is there not a clear enough evidence base to define such a target, there is also the potential to create unhelpful pressures for healthcare professionals to avoid caesareans that might promote good clinical outcomes and positive maternal experiences, as well as to undermine the decision-making power that women hold about their own births and bodies.

This is not to say that it is not beneficial to look at caesarean birth rates at all. Rather, we need a more nuanced approach, such as the widespread adoption of the Robson Group's classification system (as recommended by the World Health Organization[20]). This system enables individual trusts to look at different groups of women and assess the impact of hospital practice and policy on birth outcomes.

The diversity of caesarean birth

Not all caesarean births are the same. Some are traumatising and complex, but others are wonderful and straightforward (we'll talk much more about this in later chapters). This diversity can easily be lost in a debate that focuses solely on the overall caesarean rate. In particular, there are big differences in outcomes and maternal experience depending on the urgency of a caesarean.

The needs of women who 'need' intervention
Implicit within the debate surrounding the importance of 'medically necessary' caesareans is the notion that clinical indication is sufficient for a good overall outcome and experience for women. However, in my opinion, a 'medically necessary' caesarean is not the end of the story.

As we will see, there is much that can be done to improve the caesarean birth experience for women, including enabling truly informed decision-making, 'gentle' caesarean practices, and there is also much that can be done postnatally to support and debrief women who have either confusing or traumatic experiences. These intrapartum and postnatal needs can get lost in a debate focused on rates alone.

What is caesarean birth like in other parts of the world?

I do not have space here to present a truly meaningful and nuanced picture of caesarean birth on a global scale. Rather I want to give an overview of the global context for caesarean birth, as I believe it helps us to see more clearly the challenges surrounding improving maternal health.

Each year approximately 18.5 million caesareans are performed around the world.[21] Globally, it is estimated that the caesarean birth rate is 15%.[22] However, caesarean birth is in no way equally distributed across all communities and among all women.

Who has too little access to caesarean birth?
Women living in places that have minimal infrastructure

(particularly roads and public transportation, but also sanitation) and healthcare provision (the availability of sterile surgical equipment, anaesthetics and antibiotics), often have very little meaningful access to caesarean birth.

Globally, an estimated 289,000 women died during pregnancy and childbirth in 2013; this has declined by 45% from levels in 1990,[23] but remains a hugely significant and largely preventable loss. This reduction has been the result of a 15-year international effort to both reduce maternal mortality and increase the proportion of births that are attended by a skilled healthcare professional. But as the table below shows, there is still a lot of work to be done.

WHO region	Births attended by a skilled HCP (2007-14)[24]	Maternal Mortality Rate (2015) per 100,000[25]	% Births by Caesarean Section (2007-14)[26]
Africa	51%	542	4%
Americas	96%	52	38%
South East Asia	68%	164	10%
Europe	98%	16	25%
Eastern Mediterranean	67%	166	22%
Western Pacific	96%	41	25%
Global	**74%**	**216**	**17%**

The World Health Organization also tracks the proportion of births by caesarean in each of its global regions, as we can see in the last column. If we look deeper, there are also wide variations within regions. In Africa, for example, where the caesarean birth rate is lowest, South Sudan has a caesarean rate of less than 1% and Mauritius has a caesarean rate of 45%. Similarly, in Europe, caesarean birth rates vary significantly, ranging from 14.8% in Iceland to 52.2% in Cyprus.[27]

Caesarean provision is not just about geographical availability. The way that healthcare provision is organised can also have a significant impact on a woman's ability to access maternity care (including caesarean birth), even in places with excellent healthcare facilities. An example of this is the American healthcare system, where until the 2010 Affordable Healthcare Act, a large proportion of women struggled to find health insurance that covered pregnancy and maternity care.[28] This is now up for debate again under the Trump administration.[29]

Who has too much access to caesarean birth?
Here we move into contested territory. How many caesareans are too many? No one really knows the answer to this question – we can only make our own value judgment. So what do we know? As discussed above, we know that there is little evidence of additional benefit (in terms of maternal and neonatal mortality) when more than 10–19% of women give birth by caesarean at a population level. However, there is also currently limited evidence of additional harm.

How many countries have a caesarean rate above this level? It has been estimated that 47.2% of World Health Organization countries have a caesarean rate above 15%, particularly countries in Latin America, the Caribbean, Europe, North America and Oceania.[30]

There appears to be a strong relationship between economic development and increasing caesarean section rates: one study found that 76% of the low-income countries, 16% of the medium-income countries, and 3% of high-income countries showed caesarean section rates between 0 and 10%. By contrast, 3% of low-income countries, 36% of medium-income countries, and 31% of high-income countries showed caesarean section rates above 20%.[31]

There is also an interesting relationship between caesarean birth and the position of women in different countries. In her book *Why Human Rights in Childbirth Matter*, Rebecca Schiller describes this phenomena thus:

> *as a mirror to society, childbirth, the attitudes to it, practices around it and experiences of women going through it, reflects the progress that has been made in advancing women's rights.*

For example, some of the countries in Europe with the lowest caesarean birth rates, notably Iceland, Finland and Sweden, also tend to be countries that rank highly in the Global Gender Gap Index.[32] It is, of course, possible that this link is coincidental, but I for one am incredibly intrigued by it.

Globally, there is an increasing awareness of human rights in childbirth. As we have seen, the international maternal health agenda (via the Millennium Development Goals of the United Nations) has previously focused only on reducing maternal mortality and increasing the proportion of women who are attended by skilled healthcare personnel in labour. However, as we move further into the now not-so-new millennium:

> *there is now a greater recognition of the importance of dignity, respect and autonomy for women who do utilise healthcare facilities... The new UN Sustainable Development Goals are far more rights based.*[33]

2

Informed Choice and Finding Your Voice

Informed choice. It must be the most commonly used phrase when discussing caesarean birth. But what is it exactly? And how can you go about making one?

1. Informed choice is your human right

The concept of informed choice redefines traditional ideas about the role of healthcare professionals in decision-making: 'in the past it used to be that a doctor tells the patient what to do and the patient has no choice but to follow.'[1] It means that:

> *Pregnant women – like everyone else – have the right to make their own decisions about their bodies. It is against the law to give medical treatment to a pregnant woman unless she agrees to it. This is known legally as giving her consent.*[2]

And what is consent?

> *For consent to 'count' in law, a person must genuinely agree to receive treatment. They must be well enough informed about the treatment, and cannot have been put under undue pressure or bullied into receiving the treatment by healthcare professionals or family members.*[3]

Assuming that you are of sound mind (which if you are reading this you very likely are), no one can force you to have a caesarean birth (or any other kind of investigation/treatment). Of course, there will be circumstances in which it may be in your (and/or your baby's) best interests to do so, but that does not negate the fact that the final decision (from a legal perspective at least) is solely in your hands.

You may feel that you are not qualified to make such a life or death decision. Of course you are! You have carried your baby (or babies) for many months to reach the point where caesarean birth is a possibility, and you will be the person living with the ongoing impact of any decision made for years to come. This means you are uniquely qualified to make all decisions that will affect your body and your baby, as well as uniquely motivated to understand the short and long-term impact of these decisions.

This is not to say that you will automatically understand all of the possible benefits and limitations of any course of action. Or that you will never look to your caregiver for a recommendation, rather than a list of options (especially if things are happening very quickly – I hear you, I made that call too).

You are (most likely) not a qualified and experienced healthcare professional, with a medical or midwifery degree and years of experience. Luckily you don't have to be. It is your caregivers' role to give you accurate information about the individual risks that apply to your pregnancy and birth, mostly before a caesarean takes place, but sometimes afterwards.

In a nutshell, informed choice (or consent) affirms that *it is your body and you are the only person who can (and should) make decisions about what happens to it*.[4] The information that you are given to help you make a decision should include not only the benefits and limitations of the option that your healthcare professional is recommending, but also the benefits and limitations of any other options (including doing nothing).

2. Informed choice is 'real' evidence-based medicine (and midwifery)

Involving us in decisions about our care is not only the right thing to do from a human rights perspective, it is at the leading edge of medical (and midwifery) thinking.

Over the past 30 years, evidence-based medicine advocates have been committed '*to making clinical practice more scientific and empirically grounded and thereby achieving safer, more consistent, and more cost-effective care.*'[5] It is this movement that we have to thank for the clinical guidelines that are now available to us.

Where to find evidence-based information about caesarean

- Cochrane Pregnancy and Childbirth: pregnancy.cochrane. org/welcome
- National Perinatal Epidemiology Unit: www.npeu.ox.ac.uk
- National Institute for Health and Care Excellence (NICE): www.nice.org.uk/guidance/conditions-and-diseases/ fertility--pregnancy-and-childbirth
- Royal College for Obstetrics and Gynaecology: www.rcog. org.uk/guidelines
- Baby Friendly Initiative: www.unicef.org.uk/babyfriendly/ news-and-research/baby-friendly-research/
- Labour pains website (OAA): www.labourpains.com

However, there is also increasing recognition of the limitations of the initial evidence-based model (including too much evidence[6] and a shift in focus from disease to risk[7]). In response to this, there is a growing movement towards 'real' evidence-based medicine based on meaningful dialogue rather than protocol. *Patient Preferences Matter*, a report published by the King's Fund in 2012, noted that '*several researchers have shown that treatment decisions change – sometimes dramatically – after populations of patients become well informed.*'[8]

What is 'real' evidence-based medicine?

- Makes the ethical care of the patient its top priority
- Demands individualised evidence in a format that clinicians and patients can understand
- Is characterised by expert judgement rather than mechanical rule-following
- Shares decisions with patients through meaningful conversations
- Builds on a strong clinician–patient relationship and the human aspects of care
- Applies these principles at community level for evidence-based public health

Source: Greenhalgh, 2014

The need for this approach in maternity care is clear, as the National Maternity Review published in 2016 notes:

We were told that women do not always feel like the choice is theirs and that too often they felt pressurised by their midwives and obstetricians to make choices that fitted their services... Above all, women wanted to be listened to: about what they want for themselves and their baby, and to be taken seriously when they raise concerns.[9]

3. Informed choice requires 'sitting with' the discomfort of uncertainty

As wonderful as informed choice is, it is important to remember that it is not always easy to achieve. We saw in Chapter 1 that there are not always clear-cut answers to the many questions that we have as women about our births. In the words of one midwife:

The woman of course wants to know 'what is best for me' and to put this in the context of her life. In reality, the answer is that often we do not know.[10]

We don't need to be afraid of this uncertainty – uncertainty exists in every aspect of our lives. Once we step into our decision-making power as women (with the support of our caregivers and advocates), uncertainty will come, but it was always there: we just didn't get to fully participate in understanding our options.

Indeed, given the same evidence, different women will make different choices. Why is this?

Attitude to uncertainty: one pregnant woman might be willing to accept a 1% chance of an adverse outcome in order to make her desired outcome more likely, while others would not.

How much they value different aspects of birth: For example, some women really want to experience labour and others much less so.[11]

The job for us, as women, is to think through our own personal relationship to uncertainty and how much any given aspect of birth matters to us, and then discuss it with our caregivers. Our answers will be intensely personal, but also fraught with the expectations of others (both family and healthcare professionals). We may find they change throughout pregnancy and birth (or from one pregnancy to another). You may start to feel more confident or more cautious. In this way, it is probably more helpful to talk about informed choices, rather than a singular informed choice. You may make an informed choice to plan a vaginal birth, then make another equally informed choice to give birth by caesarean. Or vice versa.

The job for healthcare professionals? I will use the words of midwife Jean Walker here:

The most important issue... is the ability to accept that

women may listen to all our advice and seek information from a wide range of sources, but may still make a choice we are not comfortable with. If we are not happy with her choice and are now going to set about changing her mind, why did we go through the motions of presenting a choice in the first place?[12]

4. Informed choice sits hand in hand with compassionate care

Closely related to the issue of uncertainty is the central role of compassion. We need caregivers who listen to our concerns and desires, even if they sometimes need to challenge us to consider other possibilities.

This is where relationship-based care is so central. When we get to know our midwife or consultant, they start to be able to tailor the information they give us to our priorities and our needs and crucially we are able to start to build trust. In the next section we will explore how we can develop this relationship with our caregivers, as well as what to do if we find it isn't working as well as it might.

Things that you can do to ensure that you are able to make informed choices about your pregnancy and birth

- Be confident in your human rights!
- Make use of the key sources of evidence-based information
- Talk to your caregiver about any questions or concerns you might have
- Use the uncertainty surrounding birth to help you clarify what is most important to you

---

How can I have a voice in my birth?

Milli Hill, founder of the Positive Birth Movement, encapsulates this perfectly when she writes:

> *You are allowed. You are allowed to say yes or no to any of the options offered to you. You have the full right to be the key decision-maker in what happens to you and your body and your baby during labour and birth.*[13]

In essence, having a voice in your birth is about setting boundaries. Not just with healthcare providers, but also with the people we love (our partners, parents and friends), and that random person in Tesco or at the bus stop.

It's about saying: 'No! You don't get to decide, I do.'

I am not saying that you should disagree with your caregiver's recommendations, nor that you should agree with them. I am not implying that you should say no to caesarean birth (though you may decide to), nor am I saying you should say no to vaginal birth (though you may decide to). I'm not even suggesting that it's a simple either/ or choice – in reality, there are thousands of decisions to make in pregnancy alone (not to mention birth and motherhood). Rather, I am saying that the law gives us more power in our births than many of us realise, and I encourage you to ask for the information and support that you deserve.

1. Set an intention

Why do you want to have a voice in your care? What do you want to achieve?

The answers to these questions will be different depending on where you are in your journey. If you are reading this antenatally, your intention might be to have a positive birth experience. Or you might have a specific birth in mind.

> What is a positive birth?
> - You are where you want to be.
> - Your choices are informed by reality not fear.
> - You are listened to and treated with respect and dignity.
> - You are empowered and enriched.
> - Your memories are warm and proud.
>
> *Source: www.positivebirthmovement.org*

If you are reading this postnatally, your intention might vary depending on how you feel about your birth. If you had a positive experience, you might be passionate about helping other women have positive experiences too. If you had a less than positive experience, it might mean raising your voice to ask for support to process your experience, or to make a broader change in your local or national maternity services.

Most women in the postnatal period (however they feel about their birth) will also need to ask for what they need practically and emotionally from friends, family and/or healthcare professionals (such as support to establish feeding, to recover, to debrief, or simply to sleep).

Wherever you are in your journey, it is never too early or too late to raise your voice. Whenever you do start to speak up for yourself, it will (most likely) feel scary. As Lucy Pearce writes in her wonderful book *Burning Woman*: '*we have received the invitation to step more fully into ourselves, but do not know if we dare to respond. We fear what comes next.*' [14]

2. Build a support network
Don't try to do it alone! The 'strength in numbers' cliché exists for a reason. Surrounding yourself with people who support and believe in you can make all the difference.

Who can you turn to for support? There are many, many options. It is mostly a matter of finding what works for you and your circumstances. Options include:

- *Your caregiver(s):* It might sound obvious, but they will know your local system and are best placed to help you understand what is available. They may even help you think through things you had never considered.
- *A Professional Midwifery Advocate (PMA):* PMAs are experienced, practising NHS midwives, who can support you in discussing your birthing options with your midwives or obstetricians, and negotiating care that is right for you and/or exploring your feelings about your birth.
- *A doula:* Doulas are women who 'mother the mother' throughout pregnancy, birth and the postnatal period. As Milli Hill writes: *'her role is simply to make you feel like a goddess no matter where or how you want to or have to give birth.'*[15] Find out more at: doula.org.uk
- *An Independent Midwife:* An Independent Midwife is a self-employed midwife, who belongs to the organisation IMUK. They are fully trained and qualified, but also autonomous. Find out more here: www.imuk.org.uk
- *The Positive Birth Movement:* a global network of free to attend antenatal groups, linked up by social media. Local PBM groups connect pregnant women together to share stories, expertise and positivity about childbirth. See: www.positivebirthmovement.org
- *Birthrights:* a UK-based charity that aims to improve women's experiences of pregnancy and birth by increasing respect for human rights. They offer an advice service: www.birthrights.org.uk/resources/advice-service
- *The Birth Trauma Association* is an organisation set up by 'mothers who wish to support other women who

have suffered difficult births and… offer[s] advice and support to all women who are finding it hard to cope with their childbirth experience.' Find out more here: www.birthtraumaassociation.org.uk

- *#Matexp* is a grassroots campaign to bring together the voices of everyone to improve maternity services. It is a great way to connect with others who share your passion for change and find out what others are already doing. Find out more here: www.facebook.com/groups/MatExp/ or by following the #matexp hashtag on Twitter.

- *Your local Maternity Voices Partnerships (previously MSLC)* provide an opportunity to work closely with healthcare professionals and commissioners to improve local services. Find out more here: nationalmaternityvoices.org.uk.

3. Gather inspiration about what's possible

I used to have a postcard that said: *'Never doubt that a small group of thoughtful, committed citizens can change the world; indeed, it's the only thing that ever has.'* It is a quote by Margaret Mead and believe me, if you spend enough time with the people and organisations listed above, you too will begin to believe that change is possible.

Start to collect stories of women and healthcare professionals doing amazing things to change birth for the better, whether by reading through www.tellmeagoodbirthstory.com or checking out all the amazing projects that are underway through Heart Mummy Connection: heartmummy.co.uk. Then keep this inspiration at the front of your mind and let it sustain you through the challenges that will inevitably come.

4. Look at the evidence base

Alongside inspiration, we need understanding. We need to reflect on what we want and to consider alternative perspectives and possibilities. I cannot take you through the evidence base surrounding your birth or change goals here (there are too many possibilities), but I can point you to robust information about caesarean birth, and I look at specific issues in detail later in the book.

Know that the combination of inspiration (imagining what might be possible in your care or local service) and evidence (developing a nuanced understanding of the issues at stake) is where the magic of raising your voice can be found.

5. Enter the 'arena'

So what happens next? After we have our network of support, our inspiration and our evidence? *We need to ask for what we want.*

This is what I call 'entering the arena', a term I've borrowed from Brené Brown.[16]

You might be sitting in your antenatal clinic appointment, nervously holding your birth plan ready to discuss it with your midwife. You might be asking for someone to help advocate for you. You might be attending your first Maternity Voices Partnership meeting, or you might be standing up in front of student midwives and obstetricians to tell your story.

There are many different ways to 'enter the arena' as a pregnant woman or mother, and in all of them you will likely feel a combination of fear, doubt, comparison, anxiety or uncertainty. None of these feel nice, and sometimes we may think: 'it's not worth it, it's too stressful'. We might back away from what is important to us. Indeed, sometimes this might make sense, as we know that a positive birth is best supported when we are relaxed and feel safe, and sometimes asking for what we need can make us feel scared (and much more vulnerable).

But moving through these feelings (whether during birth or afterwards), can lead us to something special. As Brené Brown notes: 'vulnerability is also the birthplace of love, belonging, joy, trust, empathy, creativity and innovation'. Thus, by not being put off by the uncomfortable feelings, and confidently and calmly asking for what we need, we can find our way to the absolute best things about birth.

6. Capture your successes

For some of us, capturing our successes after stepping into the arena is straightforward (even if the process of stepping in wasn't). We achieve our goals, we can proudly say: 'I believed I could so I did'. You may have experienced the positive birth that you dreamed of. You may have got the buy-in from your local maternity services to take forward your new project. I celebrate you! That is wonderful and the more often that this happens, the better birth will be for women and their babies.

For others, it is not so easy to capture the successes, but it is all the more important. Perhaps your birth was stressful or traumatic, perhaps you didn't feel listened to, perhaps you spoke up about your experiences and you were greeted with hostility or indifference. You might have a different story to tell – a story that says: *I believed I could, but in the end, I didn't.* I have stories like this, and so do many other women.

If this is you, it can be worthwhile to consider the concept of negativity bias – that we tend to focus on the things that go wrong, rather than the things that went right. This is not an 'all that matters is a healthy baby' argument. Not in the slightest. You do matter, and if something doesn't feel right to you, you should absolutely speak up about it.

We need to capture our successes in order to sustain us. For me, I didn't get the dream water birth that I wanted, nor did

I get unanimous support and compassion from every single caregiver that I met. *But,* I can think of four or five people who really saw (and listened to) me during my care. I got to hold my second baby in theatre, and I got to take photos of his birth. I get to write this book and share my perspective with you. These things really matter, even though they weren't my original goal.

Often we don't achieve everything we want immediately; indeed, we may not achieve it all in our lifetimes, but that doesn't mean we shouldn't try. Again I will turn to the words of Brené Brown, who says we all need someone to say to us: 'that sucked! It was totally as bad as you thought. But you were brave. Now let's get you cleaned up, because you are going back in.'

> *Remember:* even if you don't get everything that you want when you raise your voice (and sometimes you won't!), you still take everything that you learn into motherhood and into the rest of your life. We will talk more about the 'power' of giving birth later. For now though, it's important to remember how much having courage in (and after) your birth can shape the person you become.

7. Keep going…
Regardless of whether we achieve our initial goal or not, it is really important to keep raising our voices about our births long after the cord is cut. If we are to genuinely put women at the centre of birth, we need all women to stand up and tell their story. To ask for what they need or what would have helped them. We can all do this in different ways. I won't tell you how you should do this, but the more we support each other as women to make our own decisions, the easier our journeys will be.

3

Why Might a Caesarean Be Offered?

'If you don't know your choices, you don't have any.'
Diana Korte

This chapter is all about helping you feel prepared for birth. Unlike other books about pregnancy and birth, it is firmly focused on birth preparation in the context of caesarean birth (whether a caesarean birth is your plan A, B or Z).

I am conscious that there may be women from very different perspectives reading these words. Some of you may be 'resisting the pervasive cultural message that birth is inherently dangerous or scary,'[1] others might prefer 'a planned, controlled birth with the aid of a competent surgeon'[2] and many may not feel particularly strongly either way.

My aim here is to present the available evidence in as simple and as straightforward a way as possible. I deliberately don't make a judgement about what might be an informed choice for you, as I believe that there are many different ways to make informed decisions about caesarean birth. Two women with the same clinical circumstances and same information about their options might make completely different choices.

Sometimes we make active choices, and other times our circumstances – whether clinical or personal – mean there is only one option that looks in any way attractive. Either way, we need meaningful conversations with our caregivers so that we can explore all our options.[3] Most of all, we need to feel that we matter in our births.

I am also aware that preparing for caesarean birth antenatally is not clear-cut. As Courtney Key Jarecki notes in *Homebirth Cesarean*:

> *one of the biggest challenges for birth professionals is to walk the line between instilling confidence in a mother about the birthing process and conveying the very real possibility that she may require a caesarean to safely birth her baby.*[4]

However, when we successfully prepare women for caesarean birth, the rewards are huge. As one woman, who was planning a homebirth, describes:

> *because we spent so much time talking about my fears and concerns, and what was important to me, my midwives knew what I wanted when I was too distressed to verbalise it. They were able to advocate for me when I couldn't.*[5]

This is what I try to do here: to find the right words to balance encouragement with realism, while leaving the final assessment firmly in your hands.

How likely am I to have a caesarean birth?

Overall, in England almost 27% of births are via caesarean section,[6] so does that mean that you have a roughly 1 in 4 chance of having a caesarean?

The short answer is: kind of, but it's not that simple.

And the long answer? Your individual likelihood of benefitting from a caesarean birth could be much, much lower than the national average or much, much higher, depending on your individual circumstances.

It can vary from 100% for women who have 'absolute indications' for caesarean birth to less than 3–5% for healthy women who receive at least some care in labour in midwife-led settings.[7]

Self care questions
- How do I feel my pregnancy is progressing?
- What excites and scares me about vaginal birth?
- What excites and scares me about caesarean birth?
- What steps can I take to move into my birth with peace, confidence and connection?
- What possibilities am I open to?
- What questions do I need to ask?
- What boundaries do I need to set?

Below I explore the obstetrician-reported indications used in the 2001 National Sentinel Caesarean Section Audit.[8] This list is not exhaustive; there may well be other (rarer) indications for caesarean. Nonetheless, I hope this list gives a good introduction to the debates surrounding indications for caesarean, to help inform your discussions with your obstetrician and/or midwife.

What we will see is that 70% of caesareans are performed for indications that are much debated (breech, 'failure to progress', foetal distress and previous caesarean)[9]: this *does not* mean that they are automatically 'unnecessary'. By contrast, caesareans that are performed for 'absolute indications'[10] account for a smaller proportion.

Some of these indications would lead to a recommendation for a planned (pre-labour) caesarean, while other indications tend to emerge in labour (or have a very short decision to delivery interval, because of the health risks to mother or baby). If you are pregnant for the first time, you are more likely to have an in-labour caesarean. Data from the RCOG highlights that pre-labour caesarean births are much less common in first pregnancies (3.3%) than they are in subsequent pregnancies (12.7%).[11]

What I hope will become clear as you read through the indications listed below is that:

- Specific clinical factors can make a caesarean birth much more likely; *and*
- There is considerable ongoing debate about the best way to manage these factors among healthcare professionals.

You may also want to pay attention to the grades that organisations like RCOG and NICE give to their recommendations (that explain how strong the evidence for them is).[12]

Breech
This means that your baby is lying bottom or feet first in the womb, rather than the usual head-first position. In early pregnancy, it is very common for a baby to be breech. 30% of babies born before 28 weeks are breech, compared to 3% at term. Breech accounts for around 11% of caesarean births.[13]

Concern centres around the fact that the head (largest part) is delivered last, which can make birth more complicated. However, Professor Murphy notes that: '*With experienced support, the short-term risks for breech babies (neonatal mortality, serious morbidity) are probably not significantly greater than those for* [head first] *babies.*'[14] Some studies suggest long-term outcomes are similar too.[15]

NICE recommend that a planned caesarean birth is offered after offering to turn the baby (known as External Cephalic Version – ECV). To learn about the risks and contraindications of ECV see the NICE Caesarean Guideline.[16] ECV is successful

35–57% of the time in first pregnancies, and from 52–84% of the time in subsequent pregnancies.

Management of breech birth is an area of considerable discussion and debate among obstetricians and midwives. The RCOG stress that the preparedness of your caregivers (and place of birth) to effectively support breech birth makes a huge difference to its safety.[17]

Other unusual presentations (malpresentation)

Sometimes a baby is in an unusual position that is neither breech nor 'head down'. According to the Sentinel Audit, malpresentation was the primary indication in around 3.5% of caesarean births. The primary concern is the possibility of cord prolapse (see below) once labour starts and/or waters break. It may be connected to other indications such as placenta praevia. NICE doesn't make an explicit recommendation about whether caesarean should be offered. Obstetrician Andy Simm notes that: '*foetal malpresentations other than breech are infrequently encountered, and there is little evidence to guide practice*'.[18]

Multiple pregnancy

A multiple pregnancy is where a woman is pregnant with more than one baby. Multiple pregnancy is the primary indication in 1% of caesarean births. Approximately 59% of twin pregnancies are delivered by caesarean, 63% of which are unplanned.[19] Stillbirth rates are higher for multiple births (2%) than for singleton births (0.5%); similarly, neonatal deaths for multiples (2.5%) are higher than for singletons (0.3%). However, the evidence connecting caesarean to improved outcomes is uncertain.

The NICE guideline notes that it is current practice to offer a caesarean if the first twin is breech. It recommends that caesarean should *not* be routinely offered when the first twin is 'head down' (unless in a research trial).

You might worry about the likelihood of having a caesarean for the second twin after a vaginal birth for the first. This happens around 3.5% of the time.

Presumed foetal compromise

Also referred to as 'foetal distress', this is when a baby shows signs of lacking oxygen or nutrients from the placenta. Indications can include an abnormal CTG trace or intrauterine growth restriction (IUGR). It is the primary indication in 22% of caesareans.

The main concern is that a lack of oxygen to the baby (or babies) can lead to serious injury or even death for the foetus. The NICE guideline notes that foetal compromise can be an indication for an urgent caesarean. NICE does not recommend that caesarean is routinely offered to women whose babies are small for their gestational age.[20] Nor does it recommend continuous heart rate monitoring for healthy women.

The main challenge with foetal compromise lies in achieving an accurate diagnosis, and there is significant debate around different methods of monitoring and how they are interpreted. NICE notes that continuous electronic monitoring is associated with higher caesarean rates (increase of 5/1,000), without improving outcomes.[21]

Cord prolapse

This occurs when the umbilical cord comes out of the uterus with or before the presenting part of the foetus. Cord prolapse is not common (according to RCOG it occurs in 1/200 births[22]). It is the primary indication in 0.5% of caesarean births.

Cases of cord prolapse appear consistently in perinatal mortality enquiries, and one large study found a perinatal mortality rate of 91/1,000.[23] Immediate caesarean is recommended (within 15 minutes is ideal).[24] See the RCOG Green Top Guideline for further discussion.[25]

Placenta praevia
This occurs when the placenta partly or totally covers the cervix. Placenta praevia is the primary indication for about 3% of all caesareans. In women who have had previous caesarean births, the chances are higher (and increase with each caesarean). See Chapter 9 for more discussion about birth after caesarean.

Vaginal birth is usually impossible and poses significant risks to the mother. Women having a caesarean for placenta praevia are at increased risk of blood loss of greater than 1,000ml (severe haemorrhage – see below) compared with women having a caesarean for other indications.[26]

Planned caesarean should be offered if, at 36 weeks' gestation, a woman has a placenta that partly or completely covers the cervical opening. If you have placenta praevia at your 20-week scan, be assured that in 90–95% of cases the placenta will move as the uterus grows with your baby. A repeat scan at 32 (and 36 weeks if needed) can confirm.

Haemorrhage and placental abruption
Haemorrhage refers to bleeding before or during birth. Causes include: placenta praevia (see above) and placental abruption (where the placenta comes away from the uterus wall). These account for less than 2% of caesareans combined.

In 2012–14, 13 out of 81 maternal deaths were due to obstetric haemorrhage.[27] Immediate caesarean birth is appropriate where there is suspected compromise to mother or baby. Without immediate compromise, a senior obstetrician should support decision-making. See the relevant RCOG guidelines: Antepartum (before labour)[28] and Postpartum (after birth).[29]

Prolonged labour[30]
This occurs when labour is taking longer than expected once it is established. On average, first labours last 8–18 hours.

Prolonged labour is a very common reason for caesarean birth (second only to foetal distress). It accounts for over 20% of the total caesarean rate.

Longer periods in labour can increase the chance of complications for mother and baby as the process of labour tires them over time. Sometimes it can also be an indication that there are other problems in the birth (such as obstructed labour or awkward positioning), but these are very much debated. It is important to take into account the whole clinical picture rather than just timings.

NICE notes that using a partograph in labour can reduce the chance of an in-labour caesarean. It also provides guidelines for diagnosis and management of delay in labour.[31] NICE cautions against two methods of diagnosing cephalopelvic disproportion (a baby too big to fit through the pelvis), which can be associated with prolonged labour.[32]

There is considerable debate among healthcare professionals about the validity of 'prolonged labour' as an indication for caesarean.

As women one of the key things we can do is ask ourselves: *'Do I feel that this is a problem?'*

Sometimes we are exhausted or worried about our baby and glad to have options to consider; other times we are feeling OK and want support or ideas to continue without significant intervention.

Maternal medical conditions

This is a broad category, including maternal cardiac disease, HIV, hepatitis B, diabetes and blood disorders, for example thalassaemia. These are a relatively uncommon reason for caesarean birth, accounting for less than 2% of the overall rate. The causes for concern regarding maternal disease vary depending on the condition concerned. For example, with infectious diseases, the main concern is the transmission of the infection from mother to baby.[33] Some medical conditions are associated with a higher likelihood of caesarean birth; for example, diabetes in pregnancy or high BMI.[34]

NICE recommends offering a caesarean to women with HIV and genital herpes who meet specific criteria (see the guideline). Routinely offering planned caesarean birth is not recommended for mothers with other infectious diseases, particularly hepatitis B and C, nor is it recommended for women with diabetes, cardiac disease or a high BMI.

You will be offered routine screening for HIV and other infectious diseases as part of your antenatal care.

Previous caesarean

This relates to women who have had one or more caesarean births in previous pregnancies, and accounts for 13.8% of caesarean births (some will have had in-labour caesareans involving multiple indications). Uterine rupture (see below) is a particular focus for birth after caesarean (see Chapter 9 for more discussion).

The risks of planned caesarean and planned vaginal birth are similar (up to four caesareans), so NICE recommends that VBAC is supported if the woman chooses.

There is huge debate on this issue.

Maternal request

This is commonly defined as a caesarean birth without clinical indications. 7.3% of all caesareans are primarily driven by maternal preference, as reported by obstetricians, though some may have had additional indications (the data is unclear).

Women have a range of reasons for preferring caesarean birth. NICE recommends that a woman is offered a caesarean after counselling on the risks and benefits (including addressing fears).

Maternal request raises a range of ethical questions that are discussed in detail later in this chapter.

Uterine rupture

Uterine or womb rupture is a rare complication in which the uterus wall tears open. It occurs most often in labour when the uterus is under pressure and contracting. It occurs in just 2 in 10,000 pregnancies in the UK. One study found that the vast majority of cases (139/159) were in women who had previously given birth by caesarean.[35]

True uterine rupture is a grave complication of pregnancy and childbirth, and can lead to death of the baby and/ or the mother.[36] NICE and RCOG don't make specific recommendations about treatment of uterine rupture. Local protocols recommend: vaginal instrumental birth (if fully dilated) or category one caesarean (if not).

Further information and discussion can be found on the UKOSS site[37] and in local hospital guidelines.[38]

Previous poor outcome or traumatic delivery
Poor outcomes could include miscarriages, stillbirth or neonatal death, and a traumatic delivery could include any delivery that is perceived by the woman as being physically or emotionally traumatic. Together they are the primary indication in 2.6% of caesareans. The Birth Trauma Association estimates that as many as 200,000 women a year feel traumatised by their birth.

In the absence of other indications, the main concern will usually be for the emotional welfare of the mother. NICE doesn't make any specific recommendations, but it is encompassed by their broader principle of 'woman-centred' care.

You may want to consider arranging a debrief of your previous birth experiences, to help you go into your birth feeling more confident. You might also consider arranging an individual care plan if you are keen to plan for a a vaginal birth, but would feel more confident with continuity of carer.

Pre-eclampsia, eclampsia and HELLP

Pre-eclampsia is characterised by high blood pressure and protein in your urine during pregnancy. Eclamspia (fitting) and HELLP syndrome (liver disorder) are serious complications of pre-eclampsia. These conditions account for 2.3% of caesarean births. Mild pre-eclampsia affects up to 6% of pregnancies, and severe cases develop in 1–2% of pregnancies as reported on nhs.uk/conditions/pre-eclampsia.

Although most cases of pre-eclampsia cause no problems and improve soon after the baby is delivered, there's a risk of serious complications that can affect both the mother and her baby. NICE recommends that caesarean and vaginal birth are offered to women with severe hypertension, severe pre-eclampsia or eclampsia based on their clinical circumstances and the woman's preferences.[39]

You can access support at action-on-pre-eclampsia.org.uk

Chorioamnionitis

An acute inflammation of the membranes and chorion of the placenta. It accounts for 0.2% of caesarean births. It is more common in pre-term births (occurring in 40–70% of preterm births with premature membrane rupture or spontaneous labour, compared to 1–13% of term births).[40]

Adverse maternal outcomes include postpartum infections and sepsis, while adverse infant outcomes include stillbirth, premature birth, neonatal sepsis, chronic lung disease and brain injury leading to cerebral palsy and other neurodevelopmental disabilities.

It is not an indication for immediate caesarean without other obstetric indications (if antibiotic treatment is effective). Time-to-delivery after institution of antibiotic therapy has been shown to not affect morbidities.[41]

4

Is a Caesarean
Birth Right
for Me?

My only honest answer can be: I don't know. More importantly, I *can't* know if caesarean birth is right for you. Nor can your doula, midwife, obstetrician, partner or the *Daily Mail*. Why? We can only give you our opinion.[1]

Deciding whether to have a caesarean birth is a judgement that only you can make. *You* are the person who will carry the majority of the potential disadvantages of surgery or labour (as we will see below). *You* are the person best suited to weigh up the potential benefits to you and your baby.

You won't make this judgment alone, don't worry. You can ask your caregivers to explain the risks and benefits that they perceive for you and your baby. You can ask them to explain the different options available to you. You can ask them to explain the evidence base behind their recommendations (and how strong this evidence base is). You can disagree or you can agree. Or you can decide to trust your caregivers' recommendation, because you aren't sure whether you agree or not.

This section cannot replace a full and open discussion with your obstetrician and midwife – whether this happens prior to the caesarean or afterwards (in the case of very urgent caesareans). However, I do want to give a brief overview of the risks and benefits of caesarean birth, compared to vaginal birth, to help you enter that discussion from an informed position.

Let's start by looking at antenatal decision-making.

What are the advantages and disadvantages of a planned vaginal birth compared to a planned caesarean birth?

To answer this question, we can look to the NICE guidelines on caesarean.[2]

Planned mode of birth (for women with uncomplicated pregnancies and no previous caesarean section)

- Planned caesarean section may reduce the chance of the following in women:
  - Perineal and abdominal pain during birth and at three days postpartum
  - Injury to vagina
  - Early postpartum haemorrhage
  - Obstetric shock
- Planned caesarean section may increase the risk of the following in babies:
  - Neonatal intensive care unit admission
- Planned caesarean section may increase the risk of the following in women:
  - Longer hospital stay
  - Hysterectomy caused by postpartum haemorrhage
  - Cardiac arrest

However, it is important to note that NICE is currently planning to review this information, so as to ensure that it can fully encompass evidence about long-term outcomes for babies born by caesarean.[3] There is also emerging, but still very incomplete, evidence that vaginal birth probably has benefits that we don't yet understand – we will discuss this in greater detail in Chapter 9.

And what about the specific risks of each type of birth? Let's start by looking at:

The risks of caesarean birth

According to the RCOG,[4] a caesarean should be performed:

> *To secure the safest and/or quickest route of delivery in the circumstances present at the time the decision is made, where the anticipated risks to mother and/or baby of an alternative mode of delivery outweigh those of caesarean section.*

And what are these risks? Let's look at the RCOG consent guidance – the information that has been put together to help you make an informed decision if a caesarean birth is recommended for you (or if it is something that you ask for).

Type of risk	Description	Chance it will occur
Serious and affects mother	Emergency hysterectomy (surgical removal of uterus)	7-8 per 1,000 (uncommon)
	Need for further surgery at a later date (including curettage, where tissue is removed from the womb via surgical scraping)	5 per 1,000 (uncommon)
	Admission to intensive care unit (varies by reason for caesarean)	9 per 1,000 (uncommon)
	Thromboembolic disease. Formation in a blood vessel of a clot (thrombus) that breaks loose and is carried by the blood stream to plug another vessel.	4–16 per 10,000 (rare)
	Bladder injury	1 per 1,000 (rare)

	Ureteric injury – injury to the ureter (the tubes which carries urine from kidneys to the bladder)	3 per 10,000 (rare)
	Death	1 per 12,000 (very rare)
Mother in future pregnancies	Increased risk of uterine rupture during subsequent pregnancies/deliveries	2-7 per 1,000 (uncommon)
	Increased risk of stillbirth	1-4 per 1,000 (uncommon)
	Increased risk in subsequent pregnancies of placenta praevia and placenta accreta	4-8 per 1,000 (uncommon)
Frequent and affects mother	Persistent wound and abdominal discomfort in the first few months after surgery	9 per 100 (common)
	Increased chance of repeat caesarean section when vaginal delivery attempted in subsequent pregnancies	1 per 4 (very common)
	Readmission to hospital	5 per 100 (common)
	Haemorrhage (excessive blood loss)	5 per 1,000 (uncommon)
	Infection	6 per 100 (common)
Affects baby	Baby is cut during the procedure (laceration)	One to two babies per 100 (common)

RCOG also notes that there are other infrequent neonatal complications after delivery by caesarean section, including: foetal respiratory distress syndrome,[5] pulmonary hypertension,[6] iatrogenic prematurity[7] and difficulty with bonding and breastfeeding.[8] I discuss the evidence surrounding bonding and breastfeeding in greater detail in Chapter 8.

The risks above sound pretty sobering, don't they? However,

we cannot focus on the risks of caesarean birth in isolation. We must look at the risks of the alternative, so…

…what about vaginal birth?

During my research for this section, I spent a lot of time looking for a list of risks associated with vaginal birth (I was hoping for an equivalent consent guideline written by an organisation such as RCOG). Unfortunately I couldn't find one, though I am aware that many individual trusts are exploring how this information can be most effectively provided to women. I would encourage you to talk to your caregivers, who can help you apply this information to your locality and individual circumstances.

I have used the data collated by the National Maternity and Perinatal Audit[9] to illustrate the potential complications that can occur in a planned vaginal birth below:

Emergency caesarean (unplanned)
An emergency caesarean carries all of the potential risks outlined for caesareans above. The chance it will occur is 14.2% overall in Britain.

Use of instruments in delivery (forceps or a vacuum device)
This increases your likelihood of having an episiotomy and/or severe tear. You may still need a caesarean birth afterwards (we don't have clear evidence as to how likely this is). Your obstetrician will discuss the risks of an instrumental delivery with you and you can choose to decline (or request a caesarean instead). See the RCOG Operative Delivery consent guideline.[10] The chance that this will occur is 23.2% in a first pregnancy, and 5.1% in subsequent pregnancies.

Episiotomy
This is a surgical procedure in which an incision is made in

the perineum to enlarge the vaginal opening to improve foetal and maternal outcome. The intention is to prevent 3rd and 4th degree tears. The evidence surrounding the protective effect of an episiotomy is conflicting.[11] It is not compulsory and can be declined. Overall, episiotomies are performed in 22% of births in Britain. The rate ranges from 8.7% (for spontaneous births) to 86.1% (for instrumental deliveries).

3rd or 4th degree tear[12]
A tear that also involves the muscle that controls the anus – the anal sphincter – is known as a 3rd-degree tear. If the tear extends further into the lining of the anus or rectum it is known as a 4th-degree tear. The tear is usually repaired in theatre. The chances of having another tear in a future birth are increased: between 5 and 7 in 100 women who have had a 3rd- or 4th-degree tear will have a similar tear in a future pregnancy. Overall, 3.5% of births result in a 3rd- or 4th-degree tear. In spontaneous deliveries the rate is 5.3% in a first pregnancy and 1.6% in subsequent pregnancies. In instrumental deliveries it is 7.8% in a first pregnancy and 4.7% in a subsequent pregnancy.

Shoulder dystocia
This is when a baby's shoulder gets stuck or lodged inside the mother's pelvis. It can be very serious (it is linked to brachial plexus injury, asphyxiation and neonatal mortality). You can find out more in the RCOG patient leaflet.[13] It occurs in 1 in 150 births.

Pelvic floor damage
Damage to the pelvic floor during pregnancy and childbirth is very common. It varies in severity and it is important to note that pregnancy itself places a good deal of strain on the pelvic floor. Around 50% of women over 50 have pelvic floor prolapse.[14]

Postpartum haemorrhage
The NICE Caesarean guideline notes that an early postpartum haemorrhage is more likely after a planned vaginal birth. It is defined as when you lose more than 500ml (a pint) of blood within the first 24 hours after birth. It is common, affecting 5 in 100 women.[15] Also note that paradoxically caesarean birth itself is a risk factor for a postpartum haemorrhage.

Adverse outcome for the baby
The Birthplace study defines an adverse perinatal outcome as: intrapartum stillbirth, early neonatal death, neonatal encephalopathy, meconium aspiration syndrome and specified birth-related injuries including brachial plexus injury. These are significant outcomes that can lead to death or permanent injury. However, they are not limited to vaginal birth (adverse outcomes can occur in a caesarean birth too). There are 4.3 events per 1,000 births in healthy women. For 'higher risk' women it is harder to estimate as the risks will vary between women.

Making sense of risk

In some ways, both of the risk analyses above are limited. The caesarean birth risks encompass caesarean birth as a whole. They include 'crash' caesareans with less than fifteen minutes from decision to delivery, and caesareans that have been planned for weeks or even months. They include straightforward and complex caesareans, caesareans performed on healthy women and those performed on women who have complex health concerns.

Vaginal birth is not homogenous either. Sometimes it is straightforward (often referred to as 'normal') and other times it is complex (involving ventouse, forceps, an episiotomy and/ or a 3rd-/4th-degree tear). Sometimes we have one-to-one care from a midwife we know and trust, other times we might have a midwife (or several midwives) that we have never met before.

In this way, it often feels that we end up comparing apples and oranges when we compare vaginal birth to caesarean birth. This is where the strengths of 'real' evidence-based decision making (discussed in Chapter 1) are most keenly visible. We need an in-person, two-way discussion with our caregivers to help us understand the impact of our decision-making.

5

How Can
I Avoid a
Caesarean
Birth?

Thousands upon thousands of words have been written on this topic. Just Google 'avoid caesarean' and you will see. And yet… the caesarean birth rate continues to rise.

This is one of the most enduring paradoxes of caesarean birth: that relatively few women (especially first-time mothers) actively choose a caesarean, but many, many women give birth by caesarean anyway. There is thus a key contradiction at the heart of birth preparation: *your birth will unfold because of you,* and *in spite of you.*

Giving birth requires effort and dedication, and there are indeed things that you can do to increase your likelihood of having a straightforward, intervention-free birth if that is what you want (we'll explore what these are in a moment). However, there is also nothing you can do to *guarantee* a straightforward birth, even if some people insist otherwise.

Of course, a 'guaranteed straightforward birth' is not actually what most of us are after. As Milli Hill writes: *'women are not stupid. They actually WANT their choices to be narrowed, if this means that they and their baby are actually going to be safer! Of course they do!*[1] We just want to fully understand our options, feel listened to and retain our decision-making power.

Why do you want to avoid a caesarean birth?

This may seem like an unusual question: please don't be alarmed, I am not about to try to convince you that you should choose a caesarean birth instead. Rather, my aim is to look at common reasons for wanting to avoid a caesarean birth, and to provide you with some key things to consider (I do the same in the next section for women who want to request a caesarean).

I want to avoid the risks of a caesarean birth for myself and my baby

Caesarean birth is major surgery so it is important to be aware that complications can arise. It can also be beneficial to remember that there isn't one single 'best kind of birth' that will be applicable for every woman, in every situation: all birth carries a chance of complications. As counter-intuitive as it may seem, sometimes caesarean birth is birth gone right, even for those of us who started out wanting a straightforward vaginal birth.

I want to have the best possible birth experience

For many women, giving birth vaginally can be (and has been) a profoundly transformative experience. But don't forget that this can also be true of caesarean birth. I write more about birth experience in Chapter 7.

What does the evidence say about avoiding caesarean birth?

I do feel a little fraudulent writing a guide to avoiding caesarean birth when I myself have had two emergency caesareans. Indeed, many of the things that I suggest are things that I tried myself (particularly in preparation for my second birth). You might say: *well obviously they didn't work then!* You're right, sometimes they don't. Sometimes they won't. But sometimes

What does it mean to be 'low risk'?

In essence, being 'low risk' means that you are healthy and your pregnancy is straightforward. You can find a full list of the medical and obstetric factors that NICE uses to identify women who are 'higher risk' in the NICE Intrapartum Care guideline (CG 190).

During your booking appointment (at around 8 weeks), your midwife will discuss your medical and obstetric history in detail and use this information to make a recommendation about whether midwife-led or obstetric-led care might be more appropriate for you. NICE recommends midwife-led care for 'low risk' women and consultant-led care for 'higher risk' women (though you may still see a midwife for most of your appointments and you can decline either form of care).

While this risk assessment can change during your pregnancy or from one pregnancy to another, it is significant because it impacts on the recommendations regarding place of birth. In practical terms, being 'low risk' means that you will be given a full range of options about where to give birth:

- an obstetric unit (led by obstetricians, with midwife support);
- a co-located midwife-led unit (on the same site as the obstetric unit, but led by midwives);
- a freestanding midwife-led unit (in the community, led by midwives)
- a home birth (attended by midwives)

they do. And the evidence behind them is compelling enough for me to say: *Take a look and make up your own mind!*

The NICE Caesarean guideline has the following recommendations for reducing the likelihood of caesarean birth:

- Place of birth (discussed below)[2]
- Continuous support from women with or without prior training (see below)

- Offer of induction at 41 weeks[3]
- Use of a partogram to monitor labour[4]
- Involving consultant obstetricians in decision-making;[5] and
- Foetal blood sampling (if abnormal heart rate and foetal acidosis are suspected)[6]

I don't have space here to explore all of these in detail (I have included links to further information in the notes), but I do want to explore place of birth and continuous support.

Why does place of birth affect your likelihood of giving birth by caesarean?

The Birthplace study looked at birth outcomes for women considered to be 'low risk' in England depending on where they gave birth.[7] There is also a follow-up study looking at place of birth for 'higher risk' women, but I discuss this in further detail in Chapter 9 (as one of those 'higher risk' groups is women with a previous caesarean).

Birth outcome (all low-risk mothers)

The table below shows us that for healthy women, whose pregnancies are straightforward, the likelihood of having a caesarean birth if you start your care in an obstetric unit is almost four times higher than it is if you receive some care in labour at home.

	Home birth	Freestanding midwifery unit	Alongside midwifery unit	Obstetric unit
Normal birth	87.9%	83.3%	76.0%	57.6%
Intrapartum caesarean birth	2.8%	3.5%	4.4%	11.1%

There are three important things to note about this data:

1. It includes both first time and subsequent pregnancies.
2. It includes women who have 'complicating conditions' at the start of their labour,[8] and eight times as many women in the obstetric unit (2.5%) had two or more, compared to women who birthed at home (0.3%).
3. It focuses on women who have at least some care in their planned place of birth during labour (rather than actual place of birth), so if we want to make informed choices, it's important to also look at the proportion of women who are transferred to an obstetric unit if complications occur.

For first-time mothers (without complicating conditions at the start of labour):

	Home	Freestanding midwifery unit	Alongside midwifery unit	Obstetric unit
Transfer to an obstetric unit	45%	36.3%	40.2%	n/a[9]
Adverse perinatal outcome[10]	9.5/1,000 births (0.95%)	4.5/1,000 births (0.45%)	4.4/1,000 births (0.44%)	3.5/1,000 births (0.35%

For subsequent births (without complicating conditions at the start of labour):

	Home	Freestanding midwifery unit	Alongside midwifery unit	Obstetric unit
Transfer to an obstetric unit	12%	9.4%	12.5%	n/a
Adverse perinatal outcome	2.0/1,000 births (0.20%)	2.2/1,000 births (0.22%)	2.5/1,000 births (0.25%)	2.6/1,000 births (0.26%)

We can see that for first pregnancies, the chance of being transferred in labour is quite high (almost 1 in 2 for home births), but is much lower in subsequent pregnancies.

We can also see that for first-time mothers the chance of an adverse outcome is higher for home births than it is for obstetric unit births (but this trend is not present in subsequent births).

What is a transfer in labour like?

Does the idea of moving from one place to another in labour worry you? Let's explore what it's like.

Just like birth as a whole, each transfer is unique: sometimes it is urgent and often it is not. If you are in a non-hospital setting (being cared for by a midwife at home or in a freestanding midwife-led unit), your midwife will arrange an ambulance transfer to take you to hospital.

If you are already in hospital (in a midwife-led unit or in day assessment), it might be a matter of walking up the corridor (or being taken in a wheelchair or trolley, depending on your circumstances).

Data on reasons for transfer in labour is not always clear-cut, as studies use different definitions of an emergency transfer. However, Dr Richard Porter notes that 'the things that go wrong in the vast majority of labours (and this is particularly so with first labours), do so slowly or with plenty of warning, giving time for transfer'.[11]

Rachel's VBAC homebirth transfer story:[12]

It had been 13 hours of active labour, I had never worked so hard in my life, we had tried every trick in the book. There was no crisis, no emergency but I knew my baby was stuck. I agreed to transfer to the Rosie Delivery Unit. As the ambulance arrived (with more gas and air!) the pain became unbearable from the fear and adrenalin flowing through my body.

After the midwife checks I met the registrar, who gently asked: 'How can I help you Rachel?' I sobbed (I couldn't speak). I was assessed: dilation now 8cm – thanks adrenalin! – baby still high. The only option was a caesarean. The registrar read my birth plan and was happy to follow my wishes for a gentle caesarean.

For all birthplaces, the chance of an adverse outcome is less than 1% (which – using RCOG's lay terminology – is the equivalent of one person in a large street or a small village).[13]

It is also worth noting that there is variation across the country in terms of the likelihood of a caesarean birth in different NHS trusts. The RCOG Clinical Indicators project found that, after adjusting for relevant clinical and demographic risk factors, individual NHS trust rates ranged between 12.8% and 28.2% (10th percentile = 18.1%; 90th percentile = 25.7%).

This data doesn't separate out caesarean rates by place of birth (e.g. home vs FMU). However, we can see from the RCM Better Births project that proximity to all four choices for place of birth varies according to where you live: betterbirths.rcm.org.uk/map.

Where can I find out my local caesarean birth rate?

Although different hospitals' policies and procedures can impact your likelihood of having a caesarean, the overall caesarean rate is a relatively crude measure and may not be very helpful to you in your decision-making. Or at least not as helpful as other things that I suggest in this section, such as whether you can access one-to-one care (or a caseload midwife) or if midwife-led care is available. But if you are curious, you can look up your local statistics here: www.maternityaudit.org.uk/Audit/Charting/Clinical

However, remember:

- The World Health Organization warns against caesarean birth rate targets at a hospital or trust level (other factors such as the population served can influence the overall rate)
- Look at outcomes as a whole, not just caesarean birth
- There is variation within NHS trusts too, as one study hints at the relationship between caregiver and likelihood of caesarean: www.jognn.org/article/S0884-2175(17)30259-9/fulltext

---

Why does continuous support in labour affect your likelihood of caesarean birth?

Continuous support in labour is increasingly recognised as one of the most effective ways to increase your chances of having a straightforward, physiological birth (and indeed, your chances of having a positive birth in any clinical situation).

From a midwifery care point of view, NICE guidelines recommend women should be offered one-to-one care during established labour (generally accepted as 4cm dilation or more). This is where there is one midwife for every birthing woman, ensuring that you are not left alone in labour, except for short periods or at your request.

Continuous support can also be offered by women who are not hospital employees and have no personal relationship to the labouring woman (such as doulas), or by companions of the woman's choice from her social network (such as her husband, partner, mother, or friend).

Support in labour falls into four main categories:[14]

- *Emotional support:* includes presence, demonstrating an effective caring attitude, positive and calming verbal expressions and non-verbal expressions, distraction, use of humour.
- *Physical support and comfort measures:* including environmental control, encouragement of different positions and mobilisation, touch, massage, application of hot and cold packs, hygiene, hydrotherapy, promotion of urinary elimination and nourishment.
- *Information and advice:* includes listening to women's views, instruction on breathing and relaxation, information about routines, procedures and progress.
- *Advocacy:* includes assisting the women to make informed choices, being the woman's voice when required and conflict resolution.

A 2013 Cochrane review of 23 trials from 16 counties involving 15,000 women found that continuous support may enhance physiological labour processes as well as women's feelings of control and competence, and thus reduce the need for obstetric intervention.

Beyond the labour room, there is also growing recognition of the importance of continuity of care throughout the antenatal, intrapartum and postnatal periods. This is now being picked up as a policy priority in the 2015 National Maternity Review.

Women who are cared for by a midwife they know are:

- 16% less likely to lose their baby
- 19% less likely to lose their baby before 24 weeks
- 15% less likely to have regional analgesia
- 24% less likely to experience preterm birth
- 16% less likely to have an episiotomy[15]

However, delivering continuity has proven to be a challenge for providers. Despite the recommendation from NICE and the Department of Health that pregnant women should be cared for by a 'named' midwife, the 2015 CQC Maternity Survey found that only 75% of women said they were never left alone at any time when they were worried[16] and a joint survey from the NCT and WI (*Support Overdue*) found that 88% of women did not know their midwife when they went into labour.[17]

Other things that you might consider trying...

The NICE Caesarean guideline notes that the following have not been shown to impact the likelihood of a caesarean birth (although they are generally very safe and may impact other outcomes):

- walking in labour
- upright position during the second stage of labour

- water birth
- epidural analgesia during labour
- the use of raspberry leaves

The guideline also notes that there is a limited evidence base for the use of complementary therapies such as acupuncture, aromatherapy, hypnosis, herbal products,

---

How can I maximise my chances of getting continuous support from someone I know and trust in labour?

- *Ask about different models of care in your area:* some NHS trusts now use case-loading models of care (where women have a named midwife, or share care within small teams of midwives). There are also alternative providers who have been commissioned in some local areas to offer this type of care (check out: www.onetoonemidwives.org and www.neighbourhoodmidwives.org.uk)

Many models of continuity are primarily focused on 'low risk' women in midwife-led environments, but it is still worth exploring the possibilities for you, including:

- *Case-loading models for vulnerable women* (e.g. those with mental health needs) – ask if your NHS trust offers caseload midwifery to women who have additional needs or who are vulnerable. You can ask for someone to help advocate for you if necessary.
- *Hire a doula:* a doula is a lay person who is experienced in labour and birth (who has received some training and debriefing of her own experiences so that she can support informed decision-making).
- *Consider an Independent Midwife:* a fully qualified midwife, who can provide 'gold standard' continuity of care and help you understand your options, even if you are considered to be 'high risk'. They can support you in a hospital birth as an advocate too.

---

nutritional supplements, homeopathic medicines and Chinese medicines. However, the Royal College of Midwives notes that as many as 87% of women use complementary therapies and/or natural remedies during pregnancy, childbirth and postnatally.[18]

If you do decide to utilise complementary therapies, it is probably best to do so because they will support your general wellbeing, rather than with the expectation that they will achieve a specific outcome. They can be used alongside other forms of self-care, such as eating lots of fresh fruit and vegetables, keeping active, getting plenty of sleep and finding time to relax. All of these things will support your transition to motherhood, even if you don't end up with your plan A birth.

6

How Can
I Request a
Caesarean
Birth?

So, you want to ask for a caesarean before your obstetrician has recommended one for you? Aren't you a naughty girl!! (I say this with a wink). Depending on who you listen to, asking for a caesarean birth makes you either a unicorn or the new norm.

In reality you are neither unique nor universal. In the 2001 National Sentinel Audit, caesarean birth with maternal request as its primary (but not necessarily only) indication (as reported by clinicians) accounted for 7% of the overall caesarean rate (2% of overall births). It ranged between regions from 6% to 8% and between units from 2% to 27%.

What are the reasons that women choose a caesarean?

Of course, many women choose a caesarean due to one or more of the clinical indications we discussed in Chapter 4, but many have other equally valid reasons for preferring caesarean birth.

For blogger Kirsty Sharrock of Southwarkbelle.com, it's simply a matter of informed choice. She writes:

Either women's bodies are our own or they are not. Truly

supporting choice should mean supporting all informed decisions, not just those that someone other than the mother has deemed to be correct.[1]

For Robyn Wilder, it's a matter of knowing what she needs and asking for it.

I have mental-health issues... a severe panic disorder I was diagnosed with at 21. It has significantly impacted on my life – at one point, I was housebound for four years – and I'm concerned that I won't fare well, mentally, during an induced birth [due to gestational diabetes].[2]

Indeed, for most of the women that I speak to, their reasons for requesting a caesarean are very similar to the reasons women give for wanting to avoid one! For example, I regularly hear women explain that:

I have thought about the risks and benefits, and have decided that a planned caesarean birth poses fewer risks to me (and/or my baby) than a planned vaginal birth;

and/or

I feel a caesarean birth gives me the best possible chance at having a positive birth experience.

Some things to consider...
Before you make your final decision about whether to request a caesarean birth, I'd really encourage you to explore whether models of woman-centred vaginal birth might also be available to you (these vary from area to area, and according to your individual circumstances).

Nothing I want to write here is intended to dissuade you, only to give you opportunities to consider the wide range of choices available to you. Choice in birth is so much more than where and how you give birth (though these are important); it's about involvement in every decision, every examination and every treatment. I want to make sure that you can shape a vaginal birth just as much as you can shape a caesarean birth.

Things to think about include:

- *Continuity of carer* – if you know you will be cared for by someone that you have built a relationship with, this may help you feel more confident that you will be listened to and understood when in labour.
- *Debriefing your previous birth* (or other traumatic experiences) – regardless of your eventual decisions about birth, some women find it healing to have an opportunity to discuss their experiences with someone who will listen without judgement.
- *Making an individualised care plan* – your midwife may be able to support you to put together an individualised plan that addresses your individual concerns, whether you are worried about vaginal examinations, for example, or the possibility of perineal injury.

What do policymakers say?

In England and Wales, the 2011 NICE Caesarean guideline recommended that:

> *For women requesting a* [caesarean birth], *if after discussion and offer of support (including perinatal mental health support for women with anxiety about childbirth), a vaginal birth is still not an acceptable option, offer a planned CS.*

> *An obstetrician unwilling to perform a* [caesarean] *should refer the woman to an obstetrician who will carry out the CS.*

RCOG recommends that caesareans should take place 'where

the anticipated risks to mother and/or baby of an alternative mode of delivery outweigh those of caesarean section'.

Only when 'medically necessary'?
Internationally speaking, the position on 'maternal request' is quite different. The World Health Organization has recommended that caesarean sections are only performed when 'medically necessary'.

This language worries me. I prefer to frame this debate as caesarean births that are primarily about women's preferences, rather than being primarily about women's medical indications (although the two are not mutually exclusive).

Why? As I have already discussed, there is not always a clear consensus on when a caesarean birth is medically necessary. If obstetricians and midwives can acceptably disagree, why can't women? What does it say about our view of women in our society if we trust an obstetrician's opinion over the opinion of the woman directly affected?

I am particularly concerned by this statement from the World Health Organization:

> *the final responsibility for ensuring that caesarean section is performed only when necessary is with clinicians. The chief medical officer or the head of an obstetrics and gynaecology department in a hospital should review the indications for the caesareans that are performed.*[4]

Now I am all for accountability for clinicians,[5] and I am pretty sure that this is coming from a 'stop blaming women' point of view. However, when this approach filters down to individual hospitals, it reinforces a culture in which the obstetrician makes the decision and the woman's consent is obtained.

I would far prefer we talked about a culture in which recommendations are made by an obstetrician and the individual woman makes the final decision. A culture where obstetricians and midwives are accountable for their recommendations, not the final decision.

What are the objections to maternal request caesareans?

- *Balance of risks and benefits:* caesarean birth is major surgery and your caregivers want to make sure that you understand what the risks and benefits are.
- *Do no harm?* Some obstetricians feel uncomfortable about performing a caesarean where they perceive there is no benefit to the mother. This is a complex area (and I am not an expert in medical ethics), but I do feel that harm can, and does, happen to women in planned vaginal births, so I struggle to see the justification for declining a planned caesarean (especially when a woman is fully informed).
- *Cost:* within the NHS, financial constraints loom large in commissioning[6] decisions. Estimating the comparative cost of planned vaginal birth vs planned caesarean birth is not easy. Do we include claims for compensation from birth injury? Long-term physical therapy? The cost of emergency caesarean? The cost of future births?

  NICE costings suggest that the financial impact of maternal request ceasareans is relatively small.[7] However, the impact on the NHS budget in areas with the highest rates of maternal request caesareans could be significant. This would need to be balanced against the potentially increased costs of care (and compensation) for adverse outcomes if a woman's request is declined by caregivers.[8]
- *Potential public health impact:* Some commentators have drawn parallels between caesarean birth and antibiotics,

in that it is a lifesaving intervention, but the impact of using without need is unknown and could have a broader public health impact (see Chapter 9).

How can I best negotiate a caesarean?

The availability of maternal request caesareans varies across the country, depending on local policies and priorities. In response to this, Birthrights has launched a campaign to challenge these decisions.[9] They are reminding NHS trusts that individual obstetricians must talk to women on a one-to-one basis (having a two-way conversation) so that they can consider her individual circumstances.

Top tips
- *Discuss your request with your midwife as soon as possible.* This gives time for referrals to specialists to be made, if necessary.
- *Talk about all the available options.* Ask your caregivers to help you understand the evidence base behind their recommendations and alternatives. Ask them to help you apply the evidence to your individual circumstances.
- *If your request is declined,* ask your clinician(s) to clearly explain why, taking account of your individual circumstances.
- *Ask for a second opinion.* NICE recommends that you are referred to an obstetrician who is willing to accommodate you.
- *Read about finding your voice and support (see Chapter 2).* In particular, connecting with an Professional Midwifery Advocate will be very beneficial to you, as well as using the Birthrights advice service.

7

The
Surgical
Birth
Experience

Everything about a maternity theatre can feel unfamiliar, from the language used, to the way people dress, to the décor. Many of us will not be familiar with maternity theatres until we find ourselves in want or need of one. We may have seen the odd surgical birth on an episode of *Grey's Anatomy* or *ER*, but these dramatic depictions rarely do much to calm our nerves.

Thankfully, this is increasingly recognised by healthcare professionals, who are finding all sorts of innovative ways to make maternity theatres as welcoming and positive as possible. For example, the Birth Outside the Box Forum at the Royal Derby Hospital organised a 'Theatre Challenge' in October 2017, where staff were given the chance to experience how it felt to be a maternity theatre patient.[1]

In this chapter, I will try to unravel the enigma of caesarean birth. We'll start by looking at the different kinds of caesarean birth (from the most relaxed and unhurried, to the most rushed and urgent). Then we'll explore the surgery itself, step-by-step, including who is in the room with you.

In the previous chapters, we talked a lot about asking

questions as part of decision-making about your birth. In this chapter we will expand on this, by exploring the ways that you can personalise your experience of caesarean birth. We will also explore the following key choices in detail: pain relief, skin-to-skin and optimum cord clamping. There has also been lots of recent discussion about 'vaginal seeding': this is discussed in Chapter 9 where we explore the longer-term implications of caesarean birth.

Self-care questions

- What is important to me in my birth experience?
- Who do I want to support me during my birth?
- What possibilities am I open to?
- What questions do I need to ask?
- What boundaries do I need to set?

Are all caesareans the same?

Caesarean birth is not homogenous. There are vast differences between a planned caesarean and a category one (most urgent) emergency caesarean. There are vast differences between a straightforward caesarean and a caesarean that has complications. There are vast differences between a caesarean that utilises a spinal anaesthetic compared to a general anaesthetic (being 'put to sleep').[2]

As you read these words, I am sure you must be wondering: What is it really like? To answer I need to take you through the different types of caesarean birth and tell you women's stories of experiencing them.

How do we classify caesareans?

When we talk about the different kinds of caesarean birth, most people think about elective (planned) and emergency (unplanned) caesareans. However, RCOG has acknowledged that:

the traditional classification of caesarean section into 'elective' and 'emergency' is of limited value… because the spectrum of urgency that occurs in obstetrics is lost within a single 'emergency' category.[3]

Instead they have moved towards a new classification system:

Grade 1	Grade 2	Grade 3	Grade 4
Immediate	Urgent	Scheduled	Planned
Immediate threat to the life of the woman or fetus	Maternal or foetal compromise – not immediate	No maternal or foetal compromise but needs early delivery	Delivery timed to suit woman or staff

What does it feel like to have each of these kinds of caesarean birth?

Immediate caesareans (category one)

Around 2% of total births (and 8% of caesarean births) are performed due to indications that are considered to be immediately life-threatening.[4]

Hospitals often use something called a Decision to Delivery Interval (DDI) to assess how effective their unit is at responding to immediate threats to life. For a category one caesarean, the benchmark is a DDI of less than 30 minutes, but the sooner the better.

Many hospitals retain the colloquial term 'crash section' to describe the most urgent category one births, where there is a need for a much shorter DDI, requiring an immediate general anaesthetic (around 41% of category one caesareans use general anaesthetic).[5]

Wherever possible, your caregivers will begin something called intrauterine resuscitation[6] while you are prepped for theatre. This ensures that your baby gets as much oxygen as possible and helps to prevent any adverse impacts on them. It can also increase the time available for transfer and/or anaesthetic administration.

Depending on your individual clinical circumstances, this might include:

- Reducing contractions (either by turning off any medications that are increasing your contractions or by administering medications to halt contractions);
- Asking you to lie on your left-hand side (you'll stay in this position during the transition to theatre);
- Administering oxygen (via a mask) and IV fluids; and/or
- Treating low blood pressure (if required).
- If you are not already wearing a hospital gown, you will be supported to undress in preparation for surgery.
- Your caregivers will also reassess the clinical situation when you arrive in theatre (e.g. foetal heart rate).

The transfer to theatre during a category one caesarean is likely to be a stressful experience for all involved: woman, baby (or babies), partner and healthcare professionals. I include below some stories from women who have given birth this way.

Some women describe their experience positively:

In spite of the circumstances, (suspected foetal compromise) the staff were incredibly supportive.

In the midst of frantic activity, I remember my anaesthetist saying to me: 'I want for you, what you want for yourself'. I had asked to stay awake for the birth and, in less than 10 words, he made me feel safe and seen.

Others highlight the stressful and bewildering side of this kind of birth:

I was taken to theatre amid chaos and panic. My son was

brought into the world just minutes after the theatre doors crashed open and his little blue body was plucked from my body just in time.[7]

It felt like a road accident, I had to completely relinquish control.

Sometimes it is impossible for healthcare professionals to talk through everything that is happening during a very urgent birth, yet it is vital that, at some point during your care, you feel 'seen' by those caring for you, and that your feelings and questions are acknowledged.

Antenatal preparation for this kind of birth is tricky, as it isn't something that we actively plan for. However, being aware that it is a possibility (however uncommon) and ensuring you have people around you who know how best to support you and are ready to advocate for you, can make a huge difference.

Moreover, this is one kind of birth where postnatal emotional support and debriefing are vital, so don't be afraid to ask for what you need (even if it is years later). We'll talk more about postnatal recovery in Chapter 8.

Urgent caesareans (category two)
Category two caesareans are still urgent. There is concern about the wellbeing of mother and/or baby, but they do not require the same immediate response as a category one caesarean.

They account for almost 1 in 3 caesareans (possibly more, as category 2 and 3 weren't cross-checked against clinical indications in the statistics) and a 75-minute decision to delivery interval is often used to benchmark the effectiveness of a category two caesarean. Whereas foetal distress is the primary indication in 63.2% of category one caesareans, it is the primary indication in 34.1% of category two caesareans. Another common indication for a category two caesarean is prolonged labour (the audit used 'failure to progress', which accounted for 37% of total category two births).

One of the upsides of a category two caesarean is that there is more time to discuss the proposed mode of birth, to consider possible alternatives and to talk about ways to make it a more positive experience for all concerned (especially you!).

Everyone was calm, even though it was an emergency, they explained everything to me and made me laugh and someone in the theatre got hold of my camera and took pictures of the birth, pictures we never would have had otherwise.

It seemed like the light at the end of the tunnel after pushing with no success and almost going to an instrumental delivery.

Scheduled caesarean (category three)
A scheduled caesarean takes place when early delivery is required, but there is no immediate or urgent concern about mother or baby. In the Sentinel Audit category three caesareans accounted for 18% of caesarean births. Common indications were: prolonged labour ('failure to progress' 36.4%), breech (17.1%) and previous caesarean (13.4%).

Sometimes a woman might have been booked in for a planned caesarean but started labour early (contractions or waters breaking), or she might have been in labour for a while before choosing a caesarean over other forms of augmentation or assistance (or if these have already been attempted).

My labour started ahead of my planned caesarean section date. I was worried that because my caesarean was technically an 'emergency' that getting all my [gentle caesarean] requests met might be an issue. Thankfully, however, there was no opposition to my requests by my team on the day.

[My caesarean] was planned, but only by a few hours.

Complicated medical situation (baby's health, not mine). Birth made positive by respectful and dignified care, and kindness and compassion of the anaesthetist.

Planned caesareans (category four)
Planned caesareans are timed to suit the woman and staff. The Sentinel Audit notes that they occur when a woman is not in labour, during the daytime on a weekday. They account for approximately 31% of total caesareans.

The most common indications for this kind of caesarean are: previous caesarean (33.7%), breech (19.3%) and maternal request (18.5%).

Women tend to have very positive experiences of uncomplicated planned caesarean, particularly 'gentle' or 'woman-centred' caesarean. I asked 425 women who had had a planned caesarean whether they felt they had a positive experience and 48% rated their experience as 5/5 (most positive). This compares to more mixed experiences for women who birth by caesarean in emergency situations: 15% rated their experience as 5/5 (most positive), based on 749 responses.

I felt supported by my independent midwife and was empowered to ask all questions until I was happy with the answers. I could consider my choices. I was supported to stand my ground on decisions that I made. I felt confident in my after care choices and care of my baby.

Calm, relaxing, fully communicated to even during minor complications.

It was my choice and it was respected by all involved, I was given more information about what was going on during surgery and treated as a person. I was able to see my baby emerge as the screen was lowered and after a brief check was able to hold her skin-to-skin. The surgeons also took time to repair a lot of scar tissue and other issues left from the previous surgery and so I was mobile more quickly and recovered sooner. It was treated as a joyful experience.

Caesarean surgery: a step-by-step guide

This section looks at the whole caesarean birth process from decision-making to recovery. Of course, what I describe below might vary slightly from hospital to hospital, and from birth to birth. The steps may be condensed and/or skipped entirely, in the case of the most urgent caesareans. If this applies to you, I urge you to arrange appropriate debriefing opportunities to help you make sense of your birth experience (we will discuss this in more detail in Chapter 8). We will also talk about the ways in which you can personalise your experience.

Step one: decision-making and consent
It might seem obvious, but the first step in preparing for a caesarean birth is deciding to have one (see chapters 1 and 2). You can expect your caregivers to talk you through the reasoning behind their recommendation for caesarean birth, along with the alternative options (including doing nothing). If you have queries or concerns, don't be afraid to ask; they are there to help you feel confident in your decisions.

If you decide to proceed with a caesarean birth following this discussion, your caregiver will ask you to sign a consent form based on the information that you have been given.[8]

Step two: pre-operative appointment (planned caesareans)
If your caesarean birth is planned in advance, you will usually be invited to a pre-operative appointment (which may take place a week or two before the planned surgery). In this appointment, an appropriate healthcare professional (usually a midwife) will ensure that you are ready for surgery and help to answer any questions that you might have.

Different hospitals will have different pre-operative protocols and your caregivers' recommendations will also vary depending on your individual clinical circumstances.

The NICE Caesarean guideline recommends the following be offered to you prior to caesarean surgery:

- A blood test to check your iron levels (in case you need a transfusion during surgery)
- Prophylactic (preventative) antibiotics
- Appropriate preventative measures to avoid blood clotting, such as surgical stockings, help to walk around soon after the caesarean section, or injections during and after the operation.
- Most hospitals also have a policy of screening for MRSA prior to admission to hospital, and ask you to provide a swab sample that can be assessed.

You will be given a range of other information about where and when to arrive on the day of your surgery, who to contact if you have any questions, when to eat and drink prior to surgery and whether to use surgical soap prior to birth, as well as any medication you will need to take in advance of surgery.

Some hospitals will routinely offer to trim your pubic hair prior to surgery (using an electric razor), usually to prevent the dressing from being painful to remove postnatally. However, it is worth noting that there have been no randomised controlled trials examining this practice[9] and routine shaving is not recommended in the NICE Surgical Site Infection guideline.[10]

You will also have the opportunity to have a pre-operative discussion with your anaesthetist, who will explain your anaesthetic options and answer any of your questions.

You might want to consider asking if you can see the

operating theatre itself. Most hospitals don't offer routine tours of maternity theatres (as they are often in use, and need to be kept sterile for infection control purposes), but an increasing number of hospitals have photo or video tours on their website, or may let you have a quick peek through the door if it is not in use.

On the day itself...
On the day of the surgery, you will see a midwife to ensure you are fully prepped for surgery. This initial assessment may include:

- Checking your temperature, pulse, urine and blood pressure
- Listening to your baby's heartbeat
- Arranging an ultrasound scan (if baby is breech or if there are other concerns, such as the position of the placenta)
- Reviewing the results of your blood tests/MRSA screening

You will be given a surgical gown (or similar) to change into, as this allows for access to perform the surgery, while also protecting your privacy and dignity during the birth.

If you and your baby are well, you may find that you have to wait a while for your slot in theatre. This can be frustrating, especially as you may feel hungry, nervous about the procedure and anxious to meet your baby. However, it may comfort you a little to know that your place in the 'queue' is very often determined by the clinical indications of the other people waiting for surgery. There may not be anything you can do to speed up the process, but you can definitely ask to be kept informed and for additional advice on eating and drinking, particularly if it's likely to be a very long wait.

It may serve you best to expect a long-ish wait and then be

pleasantly surprised if you're in first. Things that might help include bringing:

- *Entertainment* (Music, a book, or your e-reader; a tablet to watch downloaded TV or movies; puzzles or colouring books). Don't forget your charger!
- *Support* (a doula, friend or partner), who can keep you company and take care of you and themselves, without eating in front of you!
- *Relaxation techniques* (it's well worth researching guided meditations, as there are tons available and if you find one that works for you it can really add to your experience).

Many mothers that I have spoken to while researching this book recommend trying to nap while you are waiting for your slot in theatre. Others go for a walk around the hospital (letting their caregivers know where they are, of course!), so you may want to hold off changing into your hospital gown if you know there will be a while to wait.

You will have different healthcare professionals come and talk to you about the planned procedure, to make sure that you feel supported, are well prepared and to give you a chance to ask any last-minute questions.

The wonderful midwife Jenny Clarke (@JennytheM) uses this waiting time to educate parents about the importance of skin-to-skin in caesarean delivery. She explains:

> *I do skin-to-skin scenarios with couples to show how I will support the mother and baby in skin-to-skin. We use a rolled up towel to mimic where baby will lie and take draft photos to get best shots lying down – all prepare for positive experience.*

You may find it helpful to talk to your midwife about skin-to-skin while you are waiting and ask for suggestions on how you can make your experience as positive as possible.

Midwife and health researcher Jeni Stevens also suggests talking to your midwife about hand-expressing while you are waiting to go into theatre. Hand-expression can help with a range of breastfeeding issues, including separation from baby, early feeding difficulties or engorgement.[12]

Who is who in theatre?[11]

There will be at least seven people looking after you in theatre (with additional people according to clinical need), including:

- **An anaesthetist,** whose role is to administer your anaesthetic and monitor your wellbeing throughout the surgery. They will stand or sit next to your head and, if you are awake, will often chat to you and your birth partner. My anaesthetist reminded my husband to take photos of our son's birth.
- **At least one Operating Department Practitioner (ODP),** who assists the anaesthetist, getting and checking the required drugs, drips or equipment.
- **At least two obstetricians.** One will be performing the surgery and the other will be assisting e.g. cutting stitches, holding instruments.
- **At least one midwife** who will support you, and your baby (once born). They will play a key role in supporting skin-to-skin while in theatre (and afterwards in recovery).
- **At least one scrub nurse or midwife** who will count all needles, stitches and instruments and hand them to the surgeon when needed.
- **A midwifery assistant or runner** to double check the swab and instrument count with the scrub midwife or nurse and 'run' to get any additional equipment required. They are not 'scrubbed up' so can go in and out of theatre to fetch things.
- **Paediatrician** who is asked to attend any 'emergency' situation, or if there are known concerns about the baby.

Step three: The surgery

While your caesarean will be a unique experience for you, your baby (or babies) and your birth partner(s), many elements of a caesarean birth are standardised to maximise the safety of you and your baby (or babies).

One of the key tools your caregivers will use to ensure your caesarean birth goes to plan is called the WHO Surgical Safety Checklist (Maternity).[13] This is a special checklist just for maternity theatres and aims to make the experience as safe as possible. The actual checklist is often tailored to local priorities and challenges, but it encompasses five key steps:

1 Briefing: The theatre team on a given day will often look at the operating list of planned surgeries for the day and discuss any potential safety problems and concerns about specific cases. For unplanned caesareans, you may hear your caregivers briefing each other about you and your circumstances as they prepare you for surgery.

2 Sign-in: When you enter theatre (either by walking yourself or on a hospital trolley), the sign-in process will take place before the anaesthetic is administered. You will be asked to confirm your name, the procedure that you are in theatre for, and whether you are happy to consent to the procedure (and any other relevant procedures that may become necessary, e.g. a blood transfusion).

The team caring for you will also confirm out loud the category of caesarean that you are having (1–4), as well as checking for allergies, known airway risks and any staffing, supplies or equipment issues (from blood products to the resuscitaire).

Once the sign-in process is completed, your anaesthetist will prepare you for your anaesthetic. We talk in detail about how this happens below.

Although this initial period can feel a little surreal, many hospitals are doing all that they can to make a caesarean birth experience as positive as possible. Obstetrician Florence Wilcock notes that '*if you lie on the operating table in the maternity theatres at my Trust you will look up and find butterflies and cherry blossom on the ceiling*.'[14] Elsewhere healthcare staff are trialling the use of light projectors to provide a more relaxing experience for expectant parents.

3 *Time out:* Once everything is prepared at the start of surgery, and before it actually begins, the team will take a 'time out' to introduce themselves to each other (name and role). They do generally know each other already, but it's standard procedure to ensure that the surgery is as safe as possible and everyone knows their role. They'll also confirm your name again. They haven't forgotten already, they are just double-checking that you are the right person for the right surgery!

Each caregiver will confirm any issues or any unusual steps that need to be taken (for example, the midwife will confirm that the catheter is draining, and the obstetrician will confirm if there are any additional procedures that are planned during the surgery).

Once this is completed the surgery itself can begin (more detail on this below).

4 *Sign-out:* Before you leave theatre, there is a final list of questions that your caregivers will run through. They will check that your baby has been labelled, and they will count all the swabs and equipment to make sure all is accounted for. All of these questions and checks are designed to ensure that your birth is as safe as humanly possible, and the process is based on international best practice.

5 *Debriefing:* The final stage is to ensure that all possible learning from the surgery is taken forward and used to improve the care

of women in the future.

While you are in recovery, each of your caregivers should speak to you to check if you have any questions or concerns. You will have opportunities to debrief your experiences with the relevant caregivers in the weeks and months afterwards (which can be particularly helpful if you have an urgent or difficult caesarean/overall birth experience).

Sources of further information
- NICE Caesarean guideline: www.nice.org.uk/guidance/cg132
- NHS Choices guide to caesarean birth: www.nhs.uk/Conditions/Caesarean-section/Pages/How-is-it-performed.aspx
- The natural caesarean: a woman-centred technique: www.ncbi.nlm.nih.gov/pmc/articles/PMC2613254

Behind the surgical drape...

Trigger warning: the text below describes the surgical process itself, so feel free to skip on if its something you'd rather not think about.

- After the go-ahead has been given, your abdomen will be cleaned. Drapes are then applied at the sides, top and bottom of your abdomen, to allow the area needed for the operation to be clearly seen. These surgical drapes will obscure your view of the surgery.
- A cut is then made into the skin across the lower part of your abdomen, down through the underlying fat until the muscles are reached. The muscles are cut down the middle and moved to the sides.
- The uterus is now visible and, like with the abdomen, a cut is made across the lower part. This will lead to the waters breaking (if they haven't already) and this fluid is suctioned out.

- Your baby is manoeuvered to allow passage through the cut in the uterus and pressure may be applied to the top of the uterus to aid delivery. Sometimes your obstetrician may use her hands or forceps to aid delivery, or may facilitate your baby to 'walk out of the womb'.
- As your baby makes their way out of the uterus, the top drape can be lowered to allow you to watch. Once delivered, you can expect to hear your baby cry after a few seconds.
- To facilitate optimum cord-clamping your baby can be placed on your thighs, where they can be dried and warmed with a towel before the cord is clamped and cut.
- If there are concerns about you or your baby, or if you are not practising optimal cord-clamping for any other reason, your obstetrician will usually clamp the cord soon after delivery and then your baby may be warmed and dried by your midwife either on your chest or at the resuscitaire.
- In many cases, you will be able to have almost immediate skin-to-skin with your baby and all checks can either wait until you are moved into recovery (e.g. weighing baby) or be undertaken while in skin-to-skin (e.g. checking baby's colour and breathing patterns).
- While you are meeting your baby, your obstetrician will remove your placenta (and may offer to preserve it for you), and will then set about sewing each layer that has been cut. Often your obstetrician will use dissolvable stitches, but sometimes s/he may use staples to close the top layers, which will need to be removed a couple of weeks later.
- A dressing is then applied on top of your abdomen.
- Now the operation is finished, you and your baby can be transferred from the operating theatre to the recovery bay. Here you will be closely monitored for a time

following the operation before being transferred to the ward).

How can I make my caesarean birth experience more positive?

Many women assume that because caesarean birth is a surgical procedure, there is little that they can do to personalise their experience. Indeed caesarean birth has been more often associated with cold and clinical surgical practices than with life-affirming rites of passage.

As we saw in the previous section, there are many aspects of a caesarean birth that are standardised and clinical – and rightly so! After all, who would want an obstetrician to lose a swab or not have best practice to rely upon in the event of complications?

However, this is yet another paradox of caesarean birth. Caesarean birth is: routine and unique; clinical and personal; and rigid and flexible.

Making a caesarean birth magical

Over the past few years, awareness of choices in caesarean birth has been growing. These choices are often grouped under different names: some talk about 'gentle'[15] caesareans or a 'natural, woman-centred technique'.[16] Others frame it as a 'Best Possible Caesarean'[17] plan or emphasise the benefits to the baby and breastfeeding by talking about a 'baby-friendly caesarean'.[18]

Whatever terminology we use, the emphasis is the same: how can we (as service users and healthcare professionals) make your caesarean birth experience more positive *for you?*

In this section, I limit my discussion to woman-centred practices. I will talk in more detail about the evidence and debates surrounding practices that potentially benefit your baby (notably vaginal seeding and optimal cord-clamping) later.

What choices can I make?

Your caesarean birth plan can be as unique as your family, but here are some ideas of what you can ask for:

- *Greater involvement in the moment of birth:* This could be by lowering the surgical drape so you can watch your baby emerge, and/or enabling your partner to video or take photos of your baby being born. Some parents choose a musical playlist to be played in theatre[19] and request that the lights are dimmed as the baby is born. Others ask that they discover the baby's sex themselves rather than being told. Some parents ask that their caregivers use homemade cord ties.[20]

- *A slower birth:* The obstetrician facilitates the baby's birth, allowing the baby to emerge on its own rather than being 'delivered', mimicking more closely a vaginal birth, and helping to compress fluid out of the baby's lungs.[21]

- *Immediate and prolonged skin-to-skin contact:* Traditionally, the baby is cleaned, weighed and dressed immediately after being born. Sometimes they are given to your partner to hold close to you, and then often taken into the recovery room while the surgery is concluded.

  Depending on your individual preferences, this traditional approach might be perfect for you. For example, if you are feeling unwell or overwhelmed, holding your baby might not feel right for you.

  With the right support from your midwife, though, skin-to-skin can transform your birth. My son, husband and I could have been the only people in the room for all I knew.

  If this appeals, you can ask your midwife to support your baby in prone position on your chest (covered with a towel to keep them warm). You can ask for all checks to take place while the baby is skin-to-skin (assuming there is no need for resuscitation) and that your baby remains with you until you are both ready to be transferred into the recovery room.

Some babies are even ready to initiate breastfeeding in theatre. Others are still sleepy from birth, but are able to enjoy the closeness with you until they are ready to feed.

Vivienne's 'gentle caesarean'

During my first pregnancy, I planned and prepared for a home birth with the utmost precision, organisation and enthusiasm, and had no reason to doubt that he would be born at home. Unfortunately, it wasn't to be, and I ended up in hospital and in need of a trip to theatre to repair a 3rd-degree tear.

Second time around, I still very much wanted a beautiful home birth, but the more practical side of me also worried for the future of my pelvic floor. I also had serious concerns about the possibility of being separated from the baby and my husband again should I need another theatre trip post-delivery – the thought can still bring tears to my eyes.

So my thoughts started to turn to elective caesarean – a world away from the birth I really wanted, but what I felt would be the safest option for my baby and me in the grand scheme of things.

Never one to go quietly, or give my health professionals an easy life, I requested a gentle caesarean. My main requests for my caesarean were that my husband was to stay with me at all times (our hospital trust usually make dads wait outside till the spinal is sited and you are ready to go), low lights, low voices, lowered drapes to watch the birth, immediate skin-to-skin and use of cord ties.

I contacted the Head of Midwifery to discuss. She was very receptive to my proposals, and went away to consult with the theatre team and my obstetrician who all reacted positively.

In the event, my labour started ahead of my planned

caesarean section date. I was worried that because my caesarean was technically an 'emergency' that getting all my requests met might be an issue. Thankfully, however, there was no opposition to my requests by my team on the day.

Once I was ready to make my way to theatre, I suddenly felt very nervous at what lay ahead – no matter how much you prepare, there is still an element of the unknown when it comes to childbirth – planned or not. Would the baby be ok? Would my husband be ok in theatre? Would I be ok? Was my baby boy at home ok? What if something went wrong?

But it was a fleeting feeling, soon replaced by excitement that in less than an hour our beautiful baby girl was going to be joining us. Who was she going to look like? How much was she going to weigh?

Once in theatre, I popped up on to the table and waited while various leads were attached to me for monitoring. I had asked for no leads to be placed on my chest to allow clear access for skin-to-skin, so they were placed on my back and ribcage instead. The clip that usually goes on a finger to measure pulse and O_2 saturation was popped on a toe. Then it was time to get my spinal, which my husband was able to support me through.

Once the surgery actually began, the atmosphere was lovely: lighthearted, yet respectful. It only felt like seconds before I was propped up a little to watch my daughter's birth. Seeing her come out of me made me feel instantly connected and she was passed – covered in vernix and shouting with great vigour – to me for immediate skin-to-skin. At that moment it could have been just us three in the theatre – I was so completely oblivious to everything else going on around me. Our little girl was here, perfect and whole, instant love filling us once again.

In under half an hour, I was through in recovery. Other than a brief five-minute cuddle with her Dad, we'd been skin-to-skin since delivery, and continued to be so. We were able *to tie off the cord with our cord ties, and my husband cut the cord. We were checked regularly, but were mainly left to bond as a family, take pictures and phone family.*

I felt high, elated, and so happy – we'd had the birth experience I'd longed for. My gentle caesarean was the healing experience I desperately needed it to be. I'm sure my fast recovery is down to how smoothly it all went and I feel very happy with my decision to go down the gentle caesarean route.

What if I have an emergency caesarean?

If you are reading this section thinking: 'that sounds lovely, but I am planning a straightforward vaginal birth and will only have a caesarean in an emergency situation, can I still make choices?' the answer is yes. In many emergency situations, there are still many ways to make your experience more positive.

- *Being aware that an urgent birth is possible can really help.* Don't panic: *possible* does not mean *probable*. The most urgent kind of caesarean (category one) is relatively uncommon, but it is by no means rare (a similar proportion of women have a category one caesarean as have a home birth – 2%).
- *Find someone to support and advocate for you in your birth.* Who you choose will vary depending on your circumstances (a doula, an Independent Midwife, your partner or your midwife).
- *Talk to them about how they can support you if urgent complications arise.* Courtney Key Jarecki (author of *Homebirth Cesarean*) encourages those supporting women to use reassuring touch, validation and narration to help ground women in their experience and prevent potential for trauma. Asking: *'what's going through your mind right now?'*

- *Write a birth plan.* What you would like if you need an urgent caesarean? Sometimes a 'slow birth' isn't possible, but skin-to-skin very often is.
- *Take it as easy as you can in the run up to your birth.* If you enter birth feeling as strong as possible, mentally and physically, you'll be best placed to be resilient to any difficulties. I know this is not always easy to do in practice (we may feel uncomfortable, have other young children to care for, or have work commitments to attend to).

What if I have a general anaesthetic?

Around 1 in 10 caesareans take place under general anaesthetic. Having a positive birth experience can be more of a challenge if you have a general anaesthetic, as you aren't awake for the birth and often it happens unexpectedly (either because you or baby are unwell, or because of problems with other anaesthetic). However, there are still things to consider and discuss with your caregivers:

- *Can my partner be in theatre?* The National Sentinel Audit found that 5% of trusts allow partners to be in theatre during a general anaesthetic caesarean, so it's not commonly allowed, but it definitely worth asking. As obstetrician Florence Wilcock notes:

Traditionally if we operate with women under a general anaesthetic (asleep), her birth partner has not been in in theatre as their role is to support the woman. Recently on several occasions, I have challenged this so that a baby is welcomed to the world with at least one of its family present and awake rather than by a group of strangers caring for the unconscious mother. There are safety considerations to be talked through for this to be successful, but it is possible. However kind and caring staff are, they are no replacement for a birth partner whom the mother has chosen to support her in the intimacy of birth.[22]

- *Will someone take photos?* Sometimes this won't be possible, as everyone is often very busy during a general anaesthetic caesarean, but there is no harm in asking (and some trusts do offer this).
- *Can someone hold my baby skin-to-skin after birth?*
- *Most of all, I am sure you will want to know what happened to your baby after birth, who held her, etc.* Ask if your midwife will record this in your notes, or ask her to talk you through it afterwards.

Helen's general anaesthetic story[23]

Helen told the Positive Birth Movement about her general anaesthetic birth plan:

I wrote down all my wishes in advance and everyone in theatre was aware that I wanted to do things a certain way. They were:

1. *Everyone uses gloves to hold my baby so she has my skin to touch first*
2. *Capture photos of everything regardless of how baby comes out*
3. *Use cord tie provided*
4. *Do not dress baby*
5. *Immediate skin-to-skin with theatre staff holding baby on me as much as possible*
6. *Neonatal checks to be done and baby put back with me*
7. *Catheter to be placed prior to GA and completely prepare me for the section prior to GA to limit GA going to baby*
8. *If needed baby to be given my expressed colostrum while I am under*
9. *Help latching baby on me as soon as possible even if I am unable to hold her*

As soon as I could after I came round from the GA, I was handed my phone and nearly burst into tears seeing the amazing photos.

My hospital is reluctant to agree to my requests...

Many of the choices outlined above are becoming much more widely available, but they are not universally practiced by all healthcare professionals in all trusts.

Here are some ideas to help you negotiate the best plan in your circumstances (see Chapter 2 for more suggestions on raising your voice):

- Write out your wishes in a birth plan (see resources box on page 85). Discuss your caesarean choices with the midwife or obstetrician who is providing your antenatal care. In this meeting:
  - Start by explaining what each of the elements of your birth plan mean to you and why you want them (e.g. you want your birth to be a life-affirming rite of passage and want to do all you can to ensure that you and baby are able to bond)
  - Then go through the plan point by point. Allow them to ask questions and, if necessary, ask them to explain the concerns they have.
  - It's important to note that while there is a study on natural caesareans underway, key elements such as skin-to-skin and optimal cord-clamping are already evidence-based.
- If you experience difficulty negotiating your wishes, you can ask for a Professional Midwifery Advocate to help you outline your needs, or you can ask to speak with the clinician in charge of caesarean guidelines and/or the Patient Advice Liaison Service.
- Stand your ground! There is really no reason for them to refuse you (assuming both you and baby are well).

Will it hurt?

No... and yes.

In the vast majority of cases, thanks to the wonders of modern anaesthetics, the surgery itself is painless and we are completely numb or unconscious during the procedure.

However, we cannot forget that caesarean birth is major surgery. It involves cutting through several layers of skin and internal tissue, which will then need time to heal. According to the NICE Caesarean guidelines, cohort studies show that 60% of women who have a caesarean (either planned or unplanned) reported having wound pain at 24 weeks after birth.[24]

Of course, pain after birth is not limited to women who birth by caesarean. While NICE notes that at three months after delivery, women who had a planned caesarean were more likely to report pain in the abdomen and pain deep inside the abdomen than women who planned a vaginal birth, they were less likely to report pain in the perineal area.

Thus it is likely that during your healing process you will experience some pain and/or discomfort. But our individual experiences vary hugely: what is slightly uncomfortable for one person, may be experienced as agony for another. The important thing to remember is that this pain can be effectively managed to support the best possible recovery.

Why is pain relief important?

Pain relief is an essential element of humane caesarean birth. Few would question the importance of pain relief during the surgery itself. Thankfully, 'natural' caesareans have nothing to do with eschewing pain-relief options.

Pain relief continues to be essential in the hours, days and weeks after birth, yet it can be more complicated to get it right. A recent Cochrane review protocol notes that:

while the women need medication to reduce the pain associated with having to sit, rise and walk relatively soon after their surgery to care for their infants, they also need to remain alert and energetic enough to interact with and breastfeed their newborns.[25]

Managing pain effectively after a caesarean has the potential to improve your overall experience of birth, as well as to contribute to long-term outcomes for yourself and your baby. Indeed, one cohort study found that severity of pain immediately after birth was associated with an increased likelihood of developing postpartum depression and persistent pain eight weeks after delivery.[26]

How likely are you to experience severe or moderate pain? On average, 50–71% of people who undergo any kind of surgery (not limited to caesarean) will experience moderate to intense pain afterwards. How intensely you experience pain will depend on your individual sensitivity and age, as well as psychological, social and environmental factors.

If you are reading this while experiencing severe pain, please talk to your midwife or health visitor about pain-relief options. You, and your needs, really matter!

Pain relief in theatre

Much of the information included below (on pages 96–102) has been taken from www.labourpains.com – a site developed by the Obstetric Anaesthetists' Association.

During your caesarean birth, you have two main options for pain relief:

- *A regional anaesthetic* (when you're awake, but completely numb in your lower body); or
- *A general anaesthetic* (when you are unconscious and have support to breathe).

Most often, a regional anesthetic is recommended during

a caesarean birth because it reduces the risk of medical complications and enables you to be involved in the birth of your baby. There are three kinds of regional anaesthetics:

- *A spinal anaesthetic* (most common, used in planned and emergency caesareans), which works by injecting anaesthetic into the fluid surrounding your spine with a very thin needle to block the nerves that carry sensations to your brain.
- *An epidural anaesthetic,* where a thin plastic tube or catheter is put next to the nerves in your backbone, and drugs to numb the nerves can be fed through the tube when needed. If you have already had an epidural sited during labour, this can be topped up with additional anaesthetic, but it does take longer than a spinal injection to work and uses more anaesthetic overall.
- *A combined spinal-epidural anesthetic or CSE* is a combination of the two. The spinal makes you numb quickly for the caesarean section. The epidural can be used to give more anaesthetic if needed, and to give pain-relieving drugs after the caesarean.

What are the benefits of regional anaesthetic?
- It is usually safer for you and your baby.
- It enables you and your partner share in the birth, and feed and hold your baby as early as possible.
- You will feel less sleepy afterwards.
- You will usually have good pain-relief afterwards.
- Your baby will usually be more alert when they are born.
- Less post-operative nausea and vomiting.

How is a regional anaesthetic administered?
Once you are in theatre, your caregivers will attach equipment to

you so that they can measure your blood pressure, heart rate, and the amount of oxygen in your blood. Your anaesthetist will then put a cannula (a thin plastic tube) into a vein in your hand or arm and will set up a drip to give you fluids.

To administer the anaesthetic, your anaesthetist will ask you to either to sit or lie on your side, and to curl your back. If you are having a planned caesarean (and sometimes for less urgent unplanned caesareans), your partner may be able to come into theatre with you while your anaesthetic is sited (offering support and reassurance). Your anaesthetist will then paint or spray your back with a sterilising solution, which feels cold, and find a suitable point in the middle of the lower back and give you a local anaesthetic injection to numb your skin. This sometimes stings for a moment.

For a spinal anaesthetic, a fine needle is put into your back. Sometimes you might feel a tingling going down one leg as the needle goes in, like a small electric shock. You should tell the anaesthetist if this happens, but try to keep as still as possible. When the needle is in the right position, they will inject local anaesthetic and a pain-relieving drug and then remove the needle. It usually takes just a few minutes, but if it is difficult to find the right spot for the needle, it may take longer.

For an epidural (or combined spinal-epidural), the anaesthetist will use a larger needle so they can place the epidural catheter (tube) into the space next to the nerves in your backbone. As with a spinal, this sometimes causes a tingling feeling or small electric shock down your leg. It is important to keep still while the anaesthetist is putting in the epidural, but once the catheter is in place they will remove the needle and you will be able to move again.

When the spinal or epidural is starting to work, your legs will begin to feel very heavy and warm. They may also start to tingle. Numbness will spread gradually up your body. The anaesthetist will check that the numbness has reached the middle of your chest before the caesarean section begins. It is sometimes necessary to change your position to make sure the anaesthetic is working well. The team will regularly take your blood pressure.

After the anaesthetist has finished putting in the spinal, epidural or combined spinal-epidural, you will be supported to lie on your back, and tilted to the left. If you feel sick at any time, you should mention this to the anaesthetist. A feeling of sickness is often caused by a drop in blood pressure. The anaesthetist can give you treatment to help this.

While the anaesthetic is taking effect, a midwife will insert a small tube (a bladder catheter) into your bladder to keep it empty during the operation. This should not be uncomfortable. The bladder catheter will usually be removed once you are able to walk and at least 12 hours after the last 'top-up dose' (a dose of spinal or epidural anaesthetic drugs given to maintain the effects of the anaesthetic). This means you won't need to worry about being able to pass urine.

What are the risks of regional anesthetic?

Scenario	How often?	Specifically
Epidural given during labour not effective enough so another anaesthetic is needed for the caesarean	Common	1/7
Spinal anaesthetic not working well enough and more drugs are needed to help with pain during the operation	Occasional	1/20
Regional anaesthetic not working well enough for caesarean and general anaesthetic is needed (spinal)	Occasional	1/50
Regional anaesthetic not working well enough for caesarean section and general anaesthetic is needed (epidural)	Occasional	1/20

Other issues include:

- It can cause itching (10–33% of the time) or a drop in blood pressure (which is easy to treat).
- It will take longer to get ready for your caesarean (important in urgent situations).
- Occasionally, it may make you feel shaky.
- You may have a tender area in the back where the needle goes in.
- You may develop a post-dural puncture headache.

What are the benefits of a general anaesthetic?

This is used less and less often nowadays, but it is sometimes needed in emergency situations (particularly category one caesareans) or in the case of maternal preference.[27] The National Sentinel Caesarean Section Audit 2001 reported that 77% of unplanned and 91% of planned caesareans used regional anesthesia.

How is a general anaesthetic administered?

In many ways, the preparation for a general anaesthetic is similar to the preparation for a regional anaesthetic. The monitoring equipment is attached to you and your anaesthetist will insert a cannula into your hand or arm.

You will be given an antacid to drink (to reduce the acid in your stomach) and a midwife may insert a catheter into your bladder before the general anaesthetic is started.

The anaesthetist will give you oxygen to breathe through a tight-fitting face mask, which they put on your face for a few minutes. Once the obstetrician and all the team are ready, the anaesthetist will put the anaesthetic in your drip to send you to sleep. Just as you go off to sleep, the anaesthetist's assistant will press lightly on your neck. This is to prevent stomach fluids getting into your lungs. The anaesthetic works very quickly.

When you are asleep, the anaesthetist will place a tube into your windpipe to allow a machine to breathe for you and also to prevent fluid from your stomach from entering your lungs. The anaesthetist will continue the anaesthetic to keep you asleep and allow the obstetrician to deliver your baby safely. But you won't know anything about any of this. The anaesthetist or obstetrician will put in some local anaesthetic which will help with the pain relief afterwards. At the end of the operation, you may be given a suppository (tablet) up your bottom to help relieve pain when you wake up.

What are the risks of general anesthetic?[28]

Type of risk	How often does this happen?	How common is it?
Chest infection	1/5	Common (most are not severe)
Sore throat	1/5	Common
Feeling sick	1/10	Uncommon
Airway problems leading to low blood-oxygen levels	1/300	Uncommon
Scratch of the eye	1/600	Uncommon
Damage to teeth	1/4,500	Rare
Awareness (being awake part of the time during your anaesthetic)	1/200–1,000	Rare
Severe allergic reaction	1/10,000–20,000	Very rare
Death	Less than 1/100,000	Very rare
Brain damage	No figures	Very rare

Pain relief in recovery

Once the caesarean birth has been completed, you may receive pain relief in a number of ways:

- You may be given a suppository (tablet) up your bottom to relieve pain when the anaesthetic wears off.
- If you've had a regional anaesthetic, the pain-relieving drugs given with your spinal or epidural should continue to give you pain relief for a few hours.
- In some hospitals, the team will leave the epidural catheter in place so they can give you more drugs later on.
- If you've had a general anaesthetic, you may be given local anaesthetic to numb some nerves in your abdomen, as well as a morphine injection or a similar painkiller.
- In some hospitals, you may be given a drip containing morphine or a similar drug. You can control the amount of painkiller you have yourself. This is called patient-controlled analgesia or PCA.

A midwife will give you tablets such as diclofenac or ibuprofen, paracetamol or morphine. It is better to take regular pain medication when nurses or doctors offer it to you than to wait until you are sore. The drugs may make you feel sleepy. Sometimes if you are breastfeeding, your baby may be affected by the pain-relieving drugs and may be a little bit sleepy too.

Pain relief at home

The NICE Caesarean guideline notes that women who have a spontaneous vaginal delivery spend on average one day in hospital, women who have an instrumental delivery spend one or two days in hospital and women who have a caesarean spend three or four days in hospital.

However, NICE also recommends that

women who are recovering well, are apyrexial [i.e. have a normal body temperature] and do not have complications following CS should be offered early discharge (after 24 hours) from hospital and follow-up at home, because this is not associated with more infant or maternal readmissions.

NICE also notes that:

There is little direct evidence to guide prescribing practice of analgesia after discharge from hospital for women who have had a [caesarean birth] with no complications. Current guidelines on [post-caesarean] wound care suggest that for mild pain paracetamol (1,000mg four times daily) should be prescribed, for moderate pain, co-codamol (one to two tablets four times daily) and for severe pain co-codamol with added ibuprofen (500mg twice daily).

If you are in pain after discharge, talk to your midwife, health visitor or GP about pain relief that might be available. If you are breastfeeding, you might find *Why Mothers' Medication Matters* by Wendy Jones helpful.[29]

Complementary medicine and pain relief

It is estimated that as many as 87% of women use complementary therapies during pregnancy, birth and the postnatal period. The evidence base surrounding non-pharmaceutical approaches to post-caesarean pain relief is still emerging. For example, researchers are currently undertaking a systematic review of aromatherapy, acupuncture, massage and music therapy. You can read about the potential benefits of each in the research protocol itself.[30]

Personally, I have found yoga to be particularly beneficial in aiding my recovery, as well as generally making me feel much better in day-to-day life. Although it is wise to ease yourself into yoga poses very gently after a caesarean, you can practice many aspects of yoga at any time (even in theatre itself!), as my favourite yoga teacher regularly reminds me: *'If you can breathe, you can practice yoga.'* If you have never tried yoga before you can find a yoga teacher who specialises in postnatal physiology and healing here: www.birthlight.co.uk. If you can't attend a class, they may be able to see you one-to-one and give you some techniques that are tailored to your recovery.

Some women swear by the benefits of 'closing the bones' massage, or seeing a chiropractor (particularly for easing back pain after birth), arnica (for reducing bruising) and peppermint tea or oil (for easing trapped wind), although these reports are anecdotal rather than evidence-based.

Dealing with trapped wind

I regularly hear people say that the most painful aspect of caesarean birth overall is trapped wind and/or constipation, and that was my experience too. A few things can help if you are suffering:

- *Chewing gum:* A Cochrane review found that *the available evidence suggests that gum-chewing in the first 24 hours after a* [caesarean] *is a well-tolerated simple, low cost, safe and easy intervention that enhances early recovery of bowel function, improves maternal comfort and potentially reduces hospital costs.*
- It is especially beneficial if eating makes you feel sick.
- *Eating lots of fruit and drinking lots of water.* After a caesarean it is very common for your bowel to be sluggish for several hours or days. This can be eased by eating foods that are easy to digest and are gentle on your healing digestive system (along with avoiding too much junk food).
- *Stool softener.* Some pain medications can also exacerbate our sluggish digestive system and can lead to constipation. You will probably be given a stool softener to help ease this and many women also swear by drinking peppermint tea.

Why should I consider skin-to-skin in theatre?

Skin to skin is a:

> *practice where a baby is dried and laid directly on their mother's bare chest after birth, both of them covered in a warm blanket and left for at least an hour or until after the first feed.*

Researchers define immediate skin-to-skin as occuring within 10 minutes of birth, and early skin-to-skin as occurring between 10 minutes and 24 hours after birth. However, the UNICEF Baby Friendly Initiative also notes that *'skin-to-skin contact can also take place any time a baby needs comforting or calming and to help boost a mother's milk supply'* (see p132).

What are the benefits of skin-to-skin?

According to the UNICEF Baby Friendly Initiative, there are a number of benefits of skin-to-skin:

- It calms and relaxes you and your baby (or babies)
- It can regulate your baby's heart rate and breathing, helping them to better adapt to life outside the womb
- It stimulates digestion and an interest in feeding
- It regulates temperature (note: NICE acknowledge that babies born by caesarean often have lower body temperatures, which may mean this is even more important)[35]
- It can enable colonisation of the baby's skin with the mother's friendly bacteria, thus providing protection against infection (see Chapter 9)
- It stimulates the release of hormones to support breastfeeding and mothering.

It is important to note that research surrounding the benefits of skin-to-skin is still ongoing, especially in the context of caesarean birth.[36] However, the evidence we have right now is compelling enough for NICE to recommend in their caesarean guideline that:

> *Early skin-to-skin contact between the woman and her baby should be encouraged and facilitated because it improves maternal perceptions of the infant, mothering skills, maternal behaviour, and breastfeeding outcomes, and reduces infant crying.*[37]

What does skin-to-skin in theatre feel like?

> *It was lovely and I'm so glad I got to experience it. Felt like it was just me and her, I was oblivious to everyone around me, in our own little bubble I loved it.* Beth

> *I think the screen was quite high up on my chest and I felt like my baby was going to roll off so the midwife cut a slit in the front of my husband's scrubs and baby roo spent his first hour or so tucked up next to daddy's chest. It was so beautiful to see and I think it was a great start to their bonding. Watching them together, knowing baby was safe, helped me relax during the rest of the surgery.* Sally

> *The lights were so bright I asked for another towel for us both to hide under – it was like no others existed while we were under our makeshift tent. I missed the rush of hormones you get with spontaneous birth but loved watching her crawl to my breast to feed. I'd asked for quiet so that I could talk to her and she responded magically to my voice.* Kimberley

> *It was amazing. I was able to breastfeed and snuggle for the duration of surgery, until they wheeled me to recovery! It made the time fly by, and they were such sweet moments. All of my anxiety was gone when she was laid on my chest!* Valerie

> *I can still remember the feel of his warm little head nestled in*

the crook of my neck, and how his little head smelled. He was quite high up due to the position of the drape, but my husband helped me hold him and it was just wonderful. Rachel

What if...

...I feel totally exhausted or unwell?

It is common for women to not feel well enough for immediate skin-to-skin in theatre or for prolonged skin-to-skin while on the postnatal ward. In theatre itself, you may experience vomiting, nausea or 'the shakes'. You may also be feeling drowsy as a result of medications during labour, or simply the physical demands that have been placed upon your body.

Many of these side-effects can be effectively managed by your anaesthetist and if you feel well enough to try skin-to-skin, be assured that your midwife will support you closely to ensure that you are both safe. Alternatively, you might ask that your partner hold your baby skin-to-skin while you rest and recover.

Once you are on the postnatal ward, skin-to-skin continues to be beneficial. However, exhaustion is a common challenge.[38] If you are struggling with looking after your baby in the hours and days after your baby is born, please do not suffer in silence. Your midwife is there to support you.

I often observe that there aren't two groups of women, those who want skin-to-skin and those who don't. I think most of us want both of these things at different times, depending on our circumstances, so that we can look after both ourselves and our babies. One of the kindest things that a maternity care assistant did for me after my second son was born was to rock him to sleep so that I could sleep for a few hours.

...I need (or choose) to have a general anaesthetic

Immediate skin-to-skin is less common in general anaesthetic caesareans, but it is not completely impossible. You can ask that your caregivers hold your baby skin-to-skin while you are unconscious (for example, read Helen's story on the Positive Birth Movement website[39]), and/or you can ask that your partner is offered the opportunity to hold your baby skin-to-skin until you regain consciousness and/or feel well enough.

...my baby is unwell and needs to be transferred to special care
The Baby Friendly Initiative notes that there are additional benefits to skin-to-skin for babies that require special care:

- It can improve oxygen saturation (oxygen in blood);
- It can reduce cortisol (stress) levels, particularly following painful procedures
- It encourages pre-feeding behaviour
- It can assist with growth
- It may reduce your baby's hospital stay

It also notes that if you express following a period of skin-to-skin contact, your milk volume will improve and the milk expressed will contain the most up-to-date antibodies.

After your caesarean, you may not be able to go with your baby to special care or the neonatal unit immediately. Your caregivers will need to balance your immediate clinical needs with your desire to be with your baby. There are two key things that you might want to consider if you want to maximise your baby's opportunities for skin-to-skin:

- You might request that your partner is able to remain with your baby (this is ideal if you also have a doula or friend to support you); and/or
- You might request that you have as many observations as possible alongside your baby. Some hospitals are experimenting with different approaches to maximising

your contact with your baby after a caesarean, so there is no harm in discussing this with your caregiver.

Optimal cord-clamping and caesarean birth

Let's start with some terminology:

- *Optimal cord-clamping* is the practice of not clamping the umbilical cord earlier than necessary (based on a clinical assessment of mother and baby). Usually it means waiting at least one minute before clamping the cord after birth.
- *Immediate cord-clamping* occurs when the cord is clamped within 30 seconds of birth, often as part of routine care.[40]
- *Deferred cord-clamping* occurs when clinicians wait at least 2–3 minutes after birth before the cord is clamped.

What are the benefits and disadvantages of waiting to clamp the cord?

A systematic review of umbilical cord clamping practices at term[41] found that:

Although early cord-clamping has been thought to reduce the risk of bleeding after birth (postpartum haemorrhage), this review of 15 randomised trials involving a total of 3,911 women and infant pairs showed no significant difference in postpartum haemorrhage rates when early and late cord-clamping (generally between one and three minutes) were compared.

There were, however, some potentially important advantages of delayed cord clamping in healthy term infants, such as higher birthweight, early haemoglobin concentration [which carries oxygen in the blood], and increased iron reserves up to six months after birth. These need to be balanced against a small additional risk of jaundice in newborns that requires phototherapy. [42]

When is immediate cord-clamping appropriate?

There are different recommendations about what accounts for clinical need. For example, the WHO states that

...early cord clamping (<1 minute after birth) is not recommended unless the neonate is asphyxiated and needs to be moved immediately for resuscitation. [43]

NICE[44] recommends that:

Women do not have the cord clamped earlier than 1 minute after the birth unless there is concern about cord integrity[45] or the baby's heartbeat. [46]

What about cord-clamping in caesarean birth?

Anecdotally, optimal cord-clamping appears to be less commonly practised during a caesarean birth, but it is entirely possible. Indeed, the WHO notes that:

The evidence base for recommendations on the optimal timing of umbilical cord-clamping for the prevention of postpartum haemorrhage includes both vaginal and caesarean births. The WHO guideline development group considered this recommendation to be equally important for caesarean sections. [47]

It is worth noting also that an RCOG paper has observed that 'placental transfusion at caesarean section appears to be less than for vaginal birth.'[48] One possible explanation focuses on the potential role of gravity on impeding blood flow from the placenta to the baby (as babies born by caesarean are lifted out of the womb and can be higher than the placenta when the cord is clamped). However, a Cochrane review found no reliable evidence to support this theory at present and recommended further research.[49] Many obstetricians will place your baby on your thighs before cutting the cord to keep baby warm and encourage maximum blood transfer.

What about cord milking/stripping?

Cord 'stripping' or 'milking' either before or after the cord is clamped has been compared with immediate cord-clamping in a number of recent trials of preterm births and of term or near-term births. There is emerging evidence that this can be beneficial, particularly for pre-term births, but at present there isn't enough evidence regarding potential harms for it to be practised routinely. If this is something you would like to consider, ask your caregiver to talk you through the potential harm vs benefit in your circumstances.

Where can I find out more about optimal cord clamping?
- NICE guidelines: www.nice.org.uk/guidance/qs105/chapter/ quality-statement-6-delayed-cord-clamping
- RCOG Impact Paper: www.rcog.org.uk/globalassets/ documents/guidelines/scientific-impact-papers/sip-14.pdf
- Full WHO Recommendations: www.who.int/elena/titles/full_ recommendations/cord_clamping/en
- Cochrane Review: onlinelibrary.wiley.com/wol1/ doi/10.1002/14651858.CD004074.pub3/abstract

What will birth be like for my partner?

First things first: when I say partner, who do I mean? I mean the person (or people) that *you* choose to accompany you during your birth. This might be your baby's father, a same-sex partner, a doula, a friend or your own mother; or a combination of the above.

Who supports you is your decision. You are not obligated

to have a particular person with you during the birth. Choose the person (or people) who will help you feel as relaxed and supported as possible. Bonus points if they encourage you to raise your voice surrounding your birth and ask for what you need.

Can your birth partner stay with you during a caesarean birth?

Yes, in most cases.

Traditionally, it has been relatively uncommon for partners to be present during a caesarean birth, but this is changing with the increased use of regional anaesthetics and increasing openness to involving partners, even during a general anaesthetic.

The 2001 National Sentinel Caesarean Section Audit noted that 89% of hospitals had guidelines about the presence of birth partners during caesarean. Of these:

- 100% facilitated the presence of birth partners when a regional anaesthetic is used (e.g. spinal or epidural); and
- 5% facilitated the presence of birth partners when a general anaesthetic is used.

What does your partner do during your caesarean birth?

Being a birth partner during a caesarean birth can be a daunting experience. The environment is often unfamiliar. They may not know what is expected of them. They may also be worried about your safety and the wellbeing of your baby (or babies).

There is also the surgery itself. In other surgical contexts, it is unusual for family and friends to be present in theatre during surgery, and it can be difficult for your birth partner to watch you being operated on.

So why do your caregivers invite your partner into theatre? They do so for two main reasons:

- *To support you.* Your birth partner probably knows you well and will often be one of your main sources of continuous support throughout your pregnancy, birth and postnatal period. They may be the only familiar face in theatre.[50]
- *To enable them to greet your baby.* Witnessing the birth of a baby can be a life-changing milestone, especially for partners who are also becoming a parent or grandparent. It can begin a lifelong bond, but it can also be a completely new, overwhelming and unfamiliar experience.

What support is available for dads and partners?

The variability of support available to dads and partners during birth is well recognised[51] and we know that giving support to others when you also need it yourself is not always easy to do.

Mark Harris, midwife and author of *Men, Love & Birth* observes that:

Too many men have left [the birth room] with mixed emotions. Often they feel very tired, both physically and mentally. Of course they are elated – witnessing the birth of your baby will be a profound experience – but these feelings of elation may be tempered by a sense of regret or shame at not being able to 'do anything' when the woman they loved seemed to need them.[52]

So what kind of support do birth partners need? No two partners are the same, but it often includes:

- *Information and advice* – to understand what is happening and why, and what is expected of them.
- *Comfort measures* – Food, drink, somewhere to sit, a change of clothes.

- *Emotional support* – acknowledgment that the birth is emotionally significant for them too, as well as appropriate avenues of additional support.

To make their experience as positive as possible, you and your partner might want to consider…

- *Hiring a doula* (or inviting another birth partner, who can share the load with your partner). Your partner might find it easier to meet his or her own physical and emotional needs when you have an extra person with you, whom you both trust. For example, your doula can look after you while your birth partner pops out to get some food if you have a long wait for your slot in theatre. A doula will also be familiar with the hospital environment and will often be able to help you navigate the system.
- *Seeking out information before your birth.* I know it can be practically difficult,[53] but if it is at all possible, it can be beneficial for your partner to attend key antenatal or pre-operative appointments, and/or antenatal classes. If possible, try to take a look at the birth environment (including theatre) ahead of time.
- *Processing their experiences.* Birth partners often do not have the same networking opportunities with other parents (due to returning to work) and may also feel reluctant to discuss their experiences.
- *Raising their voice.* A birth partner has a very different viewpoint during birth (both caesarean and vaginal). They can have an important perspective about what is and isn't working within a maternity service. (See Chapter 2)

Sources of support for partners
- *Dads Matter UK* www.dadsmatteruk.org
- *Birth Trauma Association's Dads and partners page*: www.birthtraumaassociation.org.uk/help-support/fathers-partners-page
- *Dean Beaumont's site* www.daddynatal.co.uk
- *Mark Harris's site*: www.birthing4blokes.com
- *10 top tips for caregivers*: www.nspcc.org.uk/globalassets/documents/research-reports/all-babies-count-dad-project.pdf

8

The
Postnatal
Period

As you are lifted from the operating table and onto a hospital trolley, your recovery begins. But what actually happens next?

One of the most helpful pieces of advice that my midwife gave me when she was helping me stand up after my first caesarean birth was:

> *Make sure you stand up fully (shoulders back, head up, try not to 'hunch'). It may feel uncomfortable to start with and you might want to avoid it, but it will help you heal.*

It is my hope that this chapter will help you to stand tall following your caesarean birth, both literally (to aid your physical recovery) and metaphorically (to know 'in your bones' that you have just achieved something amazing). I hope to help you navigate the immediate challenges that you will face in those first hours, days and weeks. Every caesarean recovery is different. It can be very straightforward, it can be really hard or it can be somewhere in the middle.

It might feel harder if:

- You experience a lot of pain.
- You've had a difficult or complicated pregnancy.
- You had a long labour prior to your caesarean.
- You had complications in surgery.
- You arrive on the postnatal ward at night and your birth partner is not able to stay.

It might feel easier if:

- You and/or your baby are well.
- You are supported to hold your baby skin-to-skin and initiate feeding as soon as possible (particularly if you decide to initiate breastfeeding).
- You are given compassionate and woman-centred care (antenatally, during birth and postnatally).
- Your partner or doula stays with you.
- The postnatal ward is quiet.

You may be recovering brilliantly, feeling strong and have loving support around you, or you may feel shell-shocked, exhausted and unsupported. Maybe you feel a combination of all these things. Suzanne Remic writes:

At the end of the day, your c-section is yours. Your recovery, your experience – it all belongs to you. Don't compare. Don't rush yourself. Take each day slowly, and allow yourself time to heal. You will get there, when you're ready.[1]

Self-care questions
- How am I feeling?
- What questions do I need to ask?
- What boundaries do I need to set?
- What support is available to me?
- How can I look after myself?

Your caesarean recovery step by step

In recovery
Practically speaking, the first thing that happens after your surgery is complete is that you will be taken into 'recovery'. This is usually a room that is very close to theatre, and is fully equipped and staffed to ensure that any complications can be effectively treated.

All women who are recovering from a caesarean are closely monitored to ensure that they are stable after surgery.[2] In addition, around 1 in 10 women who give birth by caesarean will require special care after their surgery (e.g. women who have had a general anaesthetic) and around 9 per 1,000 women will need intensive care.[3]

Most of the time, your baby will remain with you (or your partner if you are unwell), but if your baby is born early, or if there are other concerns about your baby's wellbeing, they may be transferred to the neonatal unit (usually on site, but sometimes they might need specialist care in another hospital).[4]

If you are well, your observations will slowly space out: starting with continuous observations if you need help to breathe and/or communicate (most often, this occurs for those who birth under general anaesthetic), moving to every 5 minutes, then every half hour, then to hourly observations. If your observations are not stable, you will be checked upon more frequently and likely reviewed by a doctor.

How can I personalise my experience?
- *Skin-to-skin* If you feel well enough, ask for support to hold your baby skin-to-skin and initiate feeding (breast or bottle). If you don't feel up to skin-to-skin (shaking and nausea can be quite common), ask if your partner can hold your baby skin-to-skin.
- *Take lots of photos* even, perhaps especially, if you think

you look awful! You don't have to show anyone else.

- *Ask questions* Each of your caregivers will come and
  see you, to check that all is well, and to let you ask any
  questions. You may find that you have lots of questions,
  but don't feel ready to ask them. That is entirely
  understandable. Do whatever feels most beneficial to you
  at that moment, and know that you can always explore
  your questions at a later date.

Arriving on the postnatal ward…

Once your caregivers are satisfied that you are stable and
there are no immediate complications, you will be taken to
the postnatal ward for further observations. They'll continue
checking your wound, temperature, blood pressure and urine
for signs of complications. They will also monitor your baby,
ensuring that they are feeding, peeing and pooing, and that
their temperature is normal.

Often the postnatal ward will consist of several bays with beds
in them (there are curtains around each bed to offer privacy).
Many hospitals also have side rooms, and have different policies
about their use. Most prioritise based on clinical needs or other
vulnerabilities (such as women who are separated from their
baby, or who have had a traumatic experience).

Most hospitals will offer you some light food as soon as
you arrive on the postnatal ward (usually tea and toast), as
long as you are stable and not feeling nauseous or vomiting.[5]
A systematic review has connected chewing gum in the early
recovery period with a speedier recovery for the gut (though
further research is needed).[6]

How can I personalise my experience?

- *Ask if you can see/stay with your baby* (if on neonatal
  unit). Some healthcare professionals will consider taking

you to see your baby on the way to the postnatal ward. If your caregivers don't offer this, there is no harm in asking. You may also be able to get some photos taken, either by your partner or by one of your caregivers. If your baby is with you, ask if you can continue to hold them while you are moved from recovery to the ward. Many hospitals will facilitate this, if it is something that you would value.

- *Ask for help to look after your baby.* You have just had major surgery and will need time to recover. Don't be afraid to use your call button (especially if your partner has been sent home).

- *Enquire about paying for a side room.* I have heard numerous women note that their trust will offer a surplus side room for an additional fee (with no guarantee of availability). I have seen prices ranging from £90 to £200 per night depending on location. The main advantage of a side room is that it can often be quieter (you will be less disturbed by people arriving on the ward, other people's babies, snoring and talking). However, it is worth bearing in mind that your own baby and monitoring can also cause sleep disturbances. The main disadvantage is that it can feel lonelier and some women prefer to be around others.

- *Ask if your birth partner can stay.* Depending on the time your baby is born, the midwives on the ward may ask your partner to leave once you arrive on the postnatal ward. Many hospitals have a policy of limiting visitors, including partners, during night-time hours. If you would like your partner or another support person to remain with you, I'd encourage you to discuss this with your caregivers antenatally and agree an appropriate plan. Likewise, if you are very uncomfortable with the idea of being on a postnatal ward with other people's partners, make sure that you discuss this too.

Regaining mobility...

Around 4–5 hours after your birth, you should start to regain mobility (if you had a spinal anaesthetic) and your midwife will help you to mobilise if you feel well enough. If you had an epidural anaesthetic, there is the option to continue the anaesthetic dose while in the postnatal ward (as an epidural can be 'topped up'). Your anaesthetist will discuss the advantages and disadvantages of this depending on your circumstances.

You will usually be encouraged to wiggle your toes and loosen your legs before being invited to sit on your bed and then stand. I would really encourage you to make sure that you stand up for the first time when your midwife or other caregiver is with you as it is common to feel lightheaded.

Once you are able to stand up and walk around (slowly to begin with!), your midwife may offer to help you have a shower or advise your partner on how to support you in doing so. You may welcome this, particularly if you had a long labour and want to freshen up, or you may not feel up to it. If you do not feel well enough to shower, you may be offered (or might want to consider requesting) a bed bath.

Around 12 hours after your last anaesthetic dose and once you are able to walk to the toilet unassisted, your midwife or a maternity care assistant will offer to remove your catheter (assuming that you are otherwise well and all observations are good). This can feel a little uncomfortable, but with a compassionate approach, where you feel relaxed, it shouldn't be painful. If you find it does hurt, do let your midwife know and she can suggest ways to make it more comfortable.

Once your catheter is removed your midwife might ask you to pee in a measuring jug or a bed pan the first few times that you use the bathroom. This is so that they can measure your output, not to check a sample of urine as they did at antenatal appointments.

Once you are comfortably eating and drinking, you can ask your midwife to remove your cannula. This can be helpful with establishing feeding, as it won't get in the way and is generally more comfortable.

NICE recommends that your wound dressing is removed after 24 hours. If you have an infection or any other issues, you may want to discuss this further with your midwife.

Your baby will also be offered several screening tests,[7] including:

- *A newborn physical examination* (within 72 hours and again at 6–8 weeks)
- *A newborn hearing screening* (often offered in hospital)
- *A newborn heel-prick test* (done at five days)

Going home

The average hospital stay after a caesarean birth is 3–4 days. However, many hospitals offer discharge as early as 24 hours after delivery, for women who are recovering well and wish to go home.

Some hospitals have 'Enhanced Recovery' pathways for women who have a planned caesarean, which are designed to facilitate earlier discharge from hospital.[8]

After discharge, a midwife (or maternity care assistant) will monitor your recovery at home, as well as checking on the progress of your baby (or babies). The frequency of these visits will be dependent on your circumstances. If you feel you need additional support, phone the number on your handheld postnatal records.

Clexane injections[9]

Most women are offered clexane injections after a caesarean birth (based on an individual risk assessment). Your midwife will offer to show you how to inject yourself and will support you (or your partner) to practise before you are discharged. These injections reduce the chance that you will develop a blood clot in your leg or lungs. They may sometimes cause bruising. You will be given a 'sharps box' in which you can safely store your used needles until your midwife can collect and dispose of them.

Looking after your wound

Around 8% of women will develop a wound infection after a caesarean birth.[10] Your likelihood of developing an infection varies based on your individual characteristics (such as BMI and age). To reduce the likelihood of infection NICE recommends the following:

- Wearing loose, comfortable clothes and cotton underwear
- Gently cleaning and drying the wound daily

Driving after a caesarean

When can I drive again after my caesarean? Getting an answer to this question can be quite frustrating! I remember asking my GP and being told: *'As soon as your insurance company says it's OK'* and asking my insurance company and being told: *'As soon as your doctor says it's OK.'*

Many use six weeks as a rule of thumb, while others suggest that it is fine to drive as soon as you feel that you can perform an emergency stop without hesitation. I'd suggest that you wait (if you can), as it will encourage you to rest as much as possible.

When should I seek medical help?

In the early days and weeks after your caesarean birth, you should receive regular visits at home from a community midwife. Initially these visits will be daily, and will then become less regular, depending on your circumstances, until you are discharged between day 10 and day 28.

During these visits, s/he will be able to provide information and advice about any concerns you might have about your or your baby's wellbeing, as well as onward referral as appropriate.

However, the NHS Choices website advises that you contact your midwife (the number should be on your postnatal notes) or GP immediately if you experience any of the following:

- severe pain
- leaking urine
- pain when peeing
- heavy vaginal bleeding
- your wound becomes more red, painful and swollen
- a discharge of pus or foul-smelling fluid from your wound
- a cough or shortness of breath
- swelling or pain in your lower leg

These symptoms may be the sign of an infection or blood clot, which should be treated as soon as possible. See: www.nhs.uk/Conditions/Caesarean-section/Pages/Recovery.aspx#pain

How can family and friends help my recovery?

The following section is written directly to your family and friends so that you can direct them to read it so that they can learn how to help you recover from your birth.

Hello family member or friend! If your partner/friend/ daughter (in law) has asked you to read this, it means that:

- You are really important to her and her baby;
- She would really value your support; *and*
- She knows how much you love, and/or care about her.

You are likely in awe of the new life that she is holding in her arms. We are never prepared, I don't think, for the powerful feelings we experience when a new baby is born.

I invite you to look at the woman who grew this life. Your partner, daughter (in law), friend. How truly wonderful is she? Her body has performed a miracle that over the past several months has required a feat of endurance, co-creation and devotion. And you now have a huge opportunity to walk this path alongside her, and deepen your relationship together.

I don't want to make assumptions about what your circumstances are, but I do want to offer you some tools that may help you on this journey (please take what resonates in your life and leave the rest).

What is it like to recover from a caesarean?
When someone has given birth by caesarean, they are healing from major abdominal surgery (the kind of surgery that would ordinarily mean no work for at least six weeks), yet almost immediately they also take on a completely new job, as primary caregiver to another, completely dependent, human being. And this is a job that they may not be fully (or even slightly) prepared for (especially if this is a first baby).

They have also just completed another 'job': growing a human being. Sharing their energy and nutrients to grow a skeleton, organs, blood and so much more. If their pregnancy or birth was complicated, they may have additional exhaustion, difficult emotions or trauma.

We also find ourselves caught in the web of modern parenting expectations, which aren't realistically achievable, even as we desperately want to do the very best for our precious baby (or babies). We may have other demands upon us: to look after other children, or other family members, to return to work to ease financial pressures, or simply to retain a sense of self in the midst of huge change.

If there is ever a time when your friend/partner/daughter (in law) needs the loving support of family and friends, it is now! But it can feel awkward to ask for help. Sometimes the 'help' that we are offered is not the 'help' that we need. Other times we might feel that we 'should' be fine, because we perceive others as 'coping better than us'.

What do women recovering from caesarean need?
Every woman is different and will need different things at different times, but I would suggest that what the vast majority of women who are recovering from birth (surgical or otherwise) need is this:

Someone to 'hold space' for them

What does it mean to 'hold space'? It means to offer support, without expectations. It means to walk alongside them as they figure out their own path, without trying to influence or control it.

This is not easy to do, especially in the context of motherhood. Most of us have formed opinions in our minds about what we would do (if we don't have kids of our own) or what was right for us (if we do), and it can be difficult for us if those we love and care about make decisions that we would not make ourselves.

But things that are hard to do are often the things that are most worth doing. Offering the help that a new mother needs, rather than the help we think she 'should' need, makes an indescribable difference. Understanding the difference takes time, patience and willingness to listen, but the rewards are incredible for your relationship with both mother and baby.

Below are some suggestions of ways in which you might support a mother who has recently had a caesarean birth:

Practical help

1. Help with daily tasks (e.g. preparing food, washing dishes, ironing clothes, cleaning or food shopping)

- Is this the best way to support her?
- What food does she like, or want, the most?
- How does she normally do these tasks (e.g. if she doesn't normally iron her socks, will doing so make her feel loved, or make her feel inadequate?)

2. Offer breastfeeding support (such as getting her snacks and drinks for long feeding sessions, helping her prop the baby with cushions, driving her to breastfeeding support sessions).

- What are her infant feeding goals?
- Remember, even if you have breastfed yourself, some of the latest advice might be different.
- See also: growingfamilies.co.uk/2016/09/21/you-make-all-the-difference-a-letter-to-the-partner-of-a-breastfeeding-mum

3. Help with baby-related tasks (changing nappies, soothing baby between feeds, learning to babywear so she can get a little sleep)
- How is she feeling about your help?
- Many new mothers will feel anxious about being separated from their baby.
- Others may be desperate for a few hours' uninterrupted rest.

4. Act as her gatekeeper

- Agree between you whether you feel up to having visitors come and meet your baby.
- If you do decide to allow visitors (and you are not obliged to), take the lead on ensuring that they are fed/watered/encouraged not to stay too long.

Emotional support

1. Listening to her talk about the birth

- She may need to tell her story repeatedly or she may not bring it up until years later.
- If you were present during the birth, think about how you want to process your own feelings about the birth.

2. 'Being' with her as she learns to mother (e.g. sitting with her during night feeds, listening to her while she talks about her worries).

- Ask her (if you are in any doubt) whether she wants empathy or solutions.
- 9 out of 10 times, empathy will be your first port of call. Put yourself in her shoes first, then you can generate better solutions together.
- You can play a key role in researching information about any questions she has. I remember being sent home from hospital with a pack of leaflets and having no time to read them.[11]

This list might feel overwhelming, but your friend or family member will often have to work through these things on her own if she isn't given support from others. There is a reason that they say 'it takes a village to raise a child'. You do not have to be the only one to help her; you can call in other reinforcements (paid or unpaid).

Don't forget: Encourage your partner/ daughter (in law)/ friend to talk to her midwife or health visitor as well. Often she may be able to access local services, such as Home-Start (www.home-start.org.uk)

What helped me (from the mouths of mothers)

My husband was amazing both times. Looked after the bigger ones, kept the house running, brought me food and drinks, let me rest unlimited amounts. Mother-in-law helped with some meals and my mum helped with school runs after hubby went back to work. Helen

I wish my husband had been given a booklet or something about support after c-section. Something that outlined physical and emotional support. I wish I could have had less visitors. I wish he could have had an extra week off work as by the time I was home from hospital he only had a week. I wish he'd known about possible emotional reactions to an emergency c-section and how to look out for warning signs of PND or PTSD. I wish he'd encouraged me to go to bed with our son, not getting dressed downstairs trying to get some sense of normality. I wish he'd known a bit more about breastfeeding. And that he'd known a bit about possible infection and painkillers. I wish he'd known about the concept of a 'baby bubble', just protecting our space at home trying to adjust. I wish he'd known about sending me back to bed to catch up on a whole week of lost sleep. I wish we'd both known about these things. Claire

I wish people know that recovery gets harder with each section! Everyone assumed I'd be used to it by number 4... Susanne

I don't understand how she's feeling...

Is your partner/friend/daughter (in law) struggling emotionally after their birth experience? Are you struggling to relate to how she is feeling? Do you want to help her feel better? Of course you do. It's painful to see someone you love hurting. But what can you do to help?

Trust her when she tells you how she feels

This is not always as easy as it might first appear, as Damon Young writes in the *Huffington Post*:

> When the concept of trust is brought up, it's usually framed in the context of actions; of what we think a person is capable of doing. If you trust someone, it means you trust them not to cheat. Or steal. Or lie. Or smother you in your sleep. By this measure, I definitely trust my wife. I trust the shit out of her.
>
> ...you know what I don't really trust?... Her feelings. If she approaches me pissed about something, my first reaction is 'What's wrong?' My typical second reaction? Before she even gets the opportunity to tell me what's wrong? 'She's probably overreacting'. My typical third reaction? After she expresses what's wrong? 'Ok. I hear what you're saying, and I'll help. But whatever you're upset about really isn't that serious.' [12]

It can be incredibly powerful to have someone you love truly hear what you are feeling. Especially in a culture that is often dismissive of women's experiences of birth (be they positive or negative).

Your partner/friend/family member may not be ready to talk to you about her feelings immediately (or indeed ever) and it is important that you respect this. But affirming that whatever they are feeling is OK, and that you are here for them whenever they need you, can leave the door open for when they are.

Will caesarean birth make it harder to bond with my baby?

First we need to ask: what do we mean by 'bonding'? Is it something that occurs only in the 'golden hour' after birth, or is it something that grows over time? Or both?

While the first hour after birth is very important (as we discussed when talking about skin-to-skin), I tend to agree with Professor Meredith Small, when she says:

Our notions of bonding have been influenced, wrongly, by research with geese. Humans are not geese, we are primates with complex social lives. Our bonding comes from time together, looking, touching, smelling, talking and getting to know our babies as they get to know us. It happens from long-term daily and nightly connections.[13]

And Vanessa Olorenshaw, who writes:

Every day since my children were born we have stitched our lives and experience together. Those repetitive moments of love, nursing, cuddles; those occasional dropped stitches of yells and tantrums and parental fails; the days where the pattern is so vibrant you wish time could stand still.[14]

Often I observe that what we are aiming for when we talk about 'bonding' is actually a much deeper concept: attachment.

the emotional bond that typically forms between infant and caregiver is the means by which the helpless infant gets primary needs met. It then becomes the engine of subsequent social, emotional and cognitive development.[15]

An older baby or young child can be said to have developed a 'secure attachment' when their mother (or other caregiver) is their 'secure base' from which to explore their environment. Attachment is not about the 'picture perfect' moments, it is about having a core relationship that offers warmth, safety, security and protection to a developing child.

There are many ways to develop a 'secure attachment' with your child (about 60% of the general population is securely attached). However, it can be hindered by life stresses that make it more difficult for parents to be responsive to their babies and children.[16] What this suggests to me is that it is absolutely vital that women are able to receive the emotional, financial, social and practical support they need after having a baby.

I am highly skeptical of the idea that caesarean birth (by itself) prevents women from developing strong attachments with their babies. The NHS appears to agree, noting:

It is unlikely that [mothers who birth by caesarean] will be any less able to bond with their baby or respond to their baby's needs than a mother that has undergone a natural delivery. [17]

Is breastfeeding possible after a caesarean birth?

In the first few days after my first caesarean I googled variations of this question whenever my son was sleeping. I was finding it difficult to establish breastfeeding as we hadn't had the best start. I found that lots of shell-shocked and overwhelmed mothers were asking the same question, as well as overwhelming reassurance that it was indeed possible.

Indeed, the NICE Caesarean guideline notes that:

Healthcare professionals caring for women who have had a CS should inform women that after a CS they are not at increased risk of difficulties with breastfeeding.

Nonetheless, there is still an abiding perception that if you have given birth by caesarean, you either can't breastfeed or you shouldn't get your hopes up.[18] So let's take a look at the data for breastfeeding after caesarean birth:

- At least 70% of women express a preference for a birth that would give them the best start to breastfeeding.[19]

- The NICE Caesarean guideline looked at randomised controlled trials that compared planned vaginal birth to planned caesarean birth and found that there was no difference in breastfeeding rates.[20]
- When looking at population-based studies that compare *actual* modes of birth the proportion of women initiating breastfeeding after a vaginal birth was higher than after a caesarean.[21] However, the studies that followed up with participants at three or six months found no difference in breastfeeding rates between vaginal birth and caesarean birth.[22]

This evidence led NICE to recommend that:

Women who have had a CS should be offered additional support to help them to start breastfeeding as soon as possible after the birth of their baby. This is because women who have had a CS are less likely to start breastfeeding in the first few hours after the birth, but, when breastfeeding is established, they are as likely to continue as women who have a vaginal birth.

What makes initiating breastfeeding easier?

- *Opting for a local anaesthetic* (spinal or epidural) rather than a general anaesthetic, if possible.
- *Immediate skin-to-skin.* Ask for your baby to be placed prone on your chest (to maximise contact) as soon as possible for as long as possible. If you are not well enough, ask your partner to do so until you are ready.
- *Asking for support.* Don't panic if things get off to a less than ideal start. It is often still possible to establish breastfeeding. Speak up and ask for help as much as you can.
- *More is more.* Feed as soon as possible and feed regularly to build your milk supply.

My breastfeeding story

When I had my first son by caesarean, I pretty much did all the things that you shouldn't. His first feed was formula, because I was exhausted and overwhelmed from trying to get him to latch, and I felt daunted by the prospect of hand-expressing (which is actually really simple once you learn the knack, at least for expressing colostrum).

My midwife helped me to latch him on for the first time the following morning (around six hours after his birth) and it was a lovely and beautiful experience. Yet I continued to have issues with latching for a couple of weeks afterwards. The main challenge was getting him into a comfortable position when my scar was still uncomfortable. I also experienced sore nipples for the first week, possibly due to awkward initial attempts to encourage my son to latch.

It was a challenging journey, especially when we found that he had lost weight at five days and needed additional monitoring. I'm not sure I would have continued if I hadn't had lots of support from my husband to help me position him, and from my midwives and health visitors, who combined close monitoring to confirm he was thriving, with reassurance that I was doing the right things to establish my milk supply.

I took it one feed, then one day, then one week at a time, never putting pressure on myself to reach the 'six months exclusive breastfeeding' milestone, which seemed a world away in those early days of round-the-clock feeding. I asked myself: 'is breastfeeding still the right choice for me today?' and gave myself permission to stop should I feel the need to.

As the weeks and then months passed, I began to feel it was easier to continue breastfeeding than it would be to stop, and ended up feeding him for 15 months.

Why have I included this story? To reassure you that (often) it can still be possible to establish breastfeeding, even if you haven't made the ideal start. I also want to stress that although we hear a lot about the benefits of breastfeeding for your baby, you really matter too.

Where can I learn more about breastfeeding?

- Ask about local breastfeeding support (both professional and peer support)
- Read about the physiology of breastfeeding:
  - *The Womanly Art of Breastfeeding* (a classic, though it encourages an attachment parenting approach, which may not be for everyone)
  - *Food of Love* by Kate Evans (an easy read with illustrations and a touch of humour)
  - *You've Got it in You* by Emma Pickett (a modern book exploring both the evidence and the challenges of breastfeeding).
- Check out helpful online sources, such as:
  - *NHS Choices* www.nhs.uk/Conditions/pregnancy-and-baby/Pages/breastfeeding-help-support.aspx
  - *KellyMom* www.kellymom.com
  - *Association of Breastfeeding Mothers* www.abm.me.uk
  - *The Breastfeeding Network* www.breastfeedingnetwork.org.uk
  - *La Leche League* www.laleche.org.uk

Did I 'give birth'?

We all feel differently about our caesarean births. You might feel that you missed something fundamental in your birth that you still long for. I hear you and I have felt that way too (or at least something similar). Alternatively, you may have a more skeptical, or even irritated, point of view. You might be thinking: *'Of course I gave birth. How dare you suggest otherwise!'* Or you may be feeling the need to both celebrate and lament. All these perspectives are valid and important.

What does it mean to 'give birth'?

According to the Oxford English Dictionary, it means: 'to bear a child or young.'[23] Mothers who birth by caesarean do this, don't they? Their baby (or babies) is (are) testament to that. A caesarean section is without doubt birth.

You are the one who grew your baby. And you are the only one who can give birth to your baby. No matter how your baby comes into the world; vaginal delivery, forceps, caesarean, you are the one who gave birth. Rachael Newman, midwife and antenatal educator

Yet many women (including myself) sometimes feel like they didn't 'give birth'. What do they mean when they say this? In my opinion, it's giving birth as power and transformation. Let's listen to the words of women:

Birth is one of the deepest and most powerful openings of any woman's life... we walk to the brink, to the edge of our courage, to the edge of the known world, and the women we thought we were. We shed our clothes, our inhibitions and our bodies open. And there in the centre of the blood and the pain, we find the women we are: deeper, stronger, more powerful, more vulnerable than we may ever have imagined. Lucy Pearce[24]

I had just experienced the most amazing thing ever! I had given birth! [this was a vaginal birth after two caesareans] There is no other experience that can compare to this. I felt physically and emotionally strong. My maternal being was in full force and I now felt complete as a woman. I had finally put Mother Nature's gift to the test and it proved to be everything I had hoped for and so much more. Michelle Quashie[25]

These are beautiful and powerful descriptions, aren't they? They are responding to the way that, in our culture,

[birth] is denied. Silenced. Ignored. Measured. Not felt. Not spoken in its fullness... Just think back to the countless times you have heard the phrase 'doctor delivers baby'... Erm, no. Mother delivers baby. Anyone else catches baby. End of chat.
Vanessa Olorenshaw[26]

Yet as mothers who birth by caesarean, reading these stories and descriptions can feel poignant, painful, and sometimes heartbreaking, or it can feel irritating and incomprehensible. We cannot describe caesarean birth as someone 'catching our baby': not in the same way, anyway. We can feel that the paths of these women are very different from our own, particularly if we feel like these very different mothers, who birthed by caesarean:

My humiliation at failing to give birth vaginally caused me to feel less than human and unworthy of love.[27]

I viewed birth merely as a means to an end and had no expectation or desire that it should be personally fulfilling or special in itself.[28]

Ironically, however, when we dig deeper we see that these stories of power and transformation through birth have much more in common with caesarean birth stories than we might think. If we take Michelle's story as an example, she talks about her journey towards a vaginal birth after two caesareans and the power of finally feeling listened to:

I sat in the room with Cathy [my consultant midwife] and the consultant and I cried! Here I was with not one but two ladies that supported my birth choice. The fear and the worry rolled down my face and away from my mind in the form of tears. I began to relax and feel safe.[29]

Similarly, Lucy notes:

If your own birthing journey was traumatic, know that it is never too late to touch the power of transformation that birth brings us. The healing may happen years after the birth itself, as you find support and witnesses to help you heal and release the energies that you could not process at the time.[30]

What I see here is that power in birth comes from embracing our vulnerability, as well as our strength. As Brené Brown writes:

...vulnerability is the core of shame and fear and our struggle for worthiness, but it appears it's also the birthplace of joy, of creativity, of belonging, of love.

However we birth, by caesarean or vaginally, we are all both vulnerable and strong.

As mothers who birth by caesarean, we accept (or request) help from others. By doing so, we are in very good company. It is rare for women to give birth without support from others and the overwhelming majority of women rely on others to hold space for us during birth (whether that is a multi-disciplinary team of healthcare professionals in theatre or a simply a partner or friend sitting in the kitchen in case we need them while birth unfolds at home).

Why do we need people to hold space for us? Because, as birthing women, we are already holding space for our babies. Mothers who birth at home need this, just as much as mothers who birth in theatre. We need partners, caregivers and advocates who walk alongside us, allowing us to be both vulnerable and strong regardless of the outcome, and who offer us unconditional support, without judgement or control.

In caesarean birth, we find power in different ways, such as:

- The power of standing in our own corner and asking for what we want (and having that power honoured).
- The power of feeling seen and supported by others (a midwife holding our babies to our chest while in theatre,

or an anaesthetist reminding our partner to take photos).

- The power of feeling heard by friends, family or healthcare professionals if we are upset or traumatised by our experiences, and hearing the vital words: *'thank you for trusting me with how you are feeling'*.
- The power of telling our story (positive or negative) so that we can empower and support other women who birth after us.

What women say:

I am strong because even though I have never shared this story publicly, I am ready to help someone else out through my experiences.[31]

I am strong because I listened to my body and had my c-section just in time to save my baby and me.[32]

Who can I talk to about how I feel?

If you need to talk to someone urgently, please contact:

- *Samaritans:* call free any time (24 hours a day, 365 days a year), from any phone on 116 123. You don't have to be suicidal to call.
- You can also call your *GP surgery* for advice. If your GP surgery is currently closed, you can use the NHS 111 service to speak to a highly trained adviser, supported by healthcare professionals.

Talking about birth can feel difficult. As Milli Hill writes:

Almost every woman who has ever given birth has a strong need to talk about it... but often in our culture, there just isn't the time or space for these conversations. Women who want to talk about how brilliant their birth was can feel awkward and worried they will upset others who had a more difficult experience. And those who had a tough time can either raise concerns – 'Do you think you are depressed?' 'Are you bonding with your baby?' – or find the opposite happens and we are silenced: 'You'll soon forget it' 'Enjoy your healthy baby'.[33]

There are also ongoing debates about the best way to talk about birth, especially difficult and/or traumatic ones, with many people raising concerns that doing so may reinforce their trauma rather than heal it.[34]

At the moment, the conclusions we can draw from the available research are limited because the available studies that explore 'postnatal debriefing' use different models, different skillsets and occur at different times in a woman's journey.

- Is it more beneficial to have a consultant debrief a woman's experience? Or a midwife? Or an interdisciplinary clinic (including anaesthetists)?
- Is it better to offer debriefing immediately after birth? Or at some point much later into their recovery?

Currently we cannot meaningfully answer these questions.

While planning a caesarean birth does not increase the likelihood of experiencing postnatal depression or PTSD compared with a planned vaginal birth,[35] we do know that birth trauma[36] and PTSD[37] are relatively common and that many of the women affected value the opportunity to talk through their births. I have met women who have asked to talk through their birth for a wide range of reasons:

- They had an urgent birth (especially if under general anaesthetic) and they want to understand what happened.
- They might have questions that they didn't feel able to ask immediately before or after their birth, but feel ready to now.
- They might be planning another birth and want to be

able to make informed choices moving forward.
- They might need closure and to have someone validate their experiences.
- They might be preparing a complaint and want to refer to their records.
- They might simply be curious to see what is written in their notes.

The right person at the right time

In the absence of a clear-cut evidence base surrounding talking about birth, it seems sensible to adopt a personalised approach, where we ask for what we need. Who we choose to talk to about our birth experiences will depend on how we are feeling and what feels most appropriate for us individually. There are a range of possibilities, including:

- *A partner (or a close friend or relative).* Those who know us well can (sometimes) be the best people to share our feelings with. This does depend upon our relationship with them. Often our family and friends may have been with us during the birth (though they may be processing their own experiences) and are ideally placed to help us recognise possible signs of postnatal depression (see box below).
- *A doula.* Many doulas will offer postnatal listening services (even if you didn't use their services for your birth). Check out doulas in your area at doula.org.uk/
- *Your midwife.* As discussed earlier in this chapter, your midwife will visit you at home (and will monitor you closely before you are discharged home). She can be an invaluable source of information and signposting to help you work through your feelings about your birth and more generally. There may also be specialist midwives

who have received training to help women explore their experiences in a safe and supported way.

- *Your health visitor.* At 10–28 days after your birth, your midwife will discharge you to health visitor care. Your health visitor will contact you to ensure you have her contact details and arrange appropriate visits. S/he can be an invaluable source of information and can often refer your for additional support.
- *Your GP.* If you prefer, you can book an appointment with your GP to discuss how you are feeling (this may be particularly appropriate if you have a long-standing relationship with them).
- A *'Birth Afterthoughts' clinic.* Many trusts offer specialist clinics where midwives, consultants and/or anaesthetists can talk through women's birth experiences and compassionately answer their questions.
- *Access to records.* You can apply to view your records at any time (they will make copies for you for a fee). Note that if you go directly to your records, you will not have a healthcare professional to talk through what they mean, or hear or validate your experience. It may be best combined with a wider discussion.
- *A counsellor.* The availability of NHS-funded counselling and/or peer support will vary from area to area. Your GP, midwife and/or health visitor should be able to advise you on local services. You can also consider paying privately. For further information see: www. birthtraumaassociation.org.uk/help-support/counsellors-therapists
- *Volunteer support*
  - *Birth Trauma Association* (www. birthtraumaassociation.org.uk or www.facebook. com/groups/TheBTA/)

- *PND and Me:* www.pndandme.co.uk/support/
- *Birth Trauma Chat* www.birthtraumatrust.org/ birthtraumachat

---

Do I have postnatal depression?

The NHS Choices website notes that possible signs of postnatal depression include:

- A persistent feeling of sadness and low mood
- Lack of enjoyment and loss of interest in the wider world
- Lack of energy and feeling tired all the time
- Trouble sleeping at night and feeling sleepy during the day
- Difficulty bonding with your baby
- Withdrawing from contact with other people
- Problems concentrating and making decisions
- Frightening thoughts – for example, about hurting your baby

See: www.nhs.uk/conditions/post-natal-depression

9

The Long-term
Impact of
Caesarean Birth

This chapter will explore the long-term impact of caesarean birth: on you, on your baby and on your future birth choices. We will start by exploring the potential long-term complications of caesarean surgery for you, with a particular focus on the potential for complications in future pregnancies. Then we will explore the longer-term outcomes for babies born by caesarean and the emerging evidence that being born this way is *associated* with long-term health problems.

It is important to note that much of the research in this area (particularly research focusing on babies born by caesarean) is still at an early stage (sometimes it is still largely hypothetical). As we saw when discussing the WHO statement on caesarean section rates in Chapter 1, the evidence surrounding the long-term impact of caesarean birth is not conclusive. NICE has not yet released its assessment of the long-term impact of caesarean birth (though it has confirmed its intention to do so).

The tentative nature of the evidence base has not diminished the wide-ranging public debates on this topic, particularly in the media. Are we really changing the face of human evolution, as some newspapers reported in 2016?[1] Often it seems that there is an awful lot of heat in these discussions, but rarely a lot of light.

However, that is not to say that we know nothing and that it is not valuable to explore what we are in the process of discovering. I will do my utmost in the pages that follow to help you digest what we know and where the gaps (and in some cases leaps of faith) are.

Self-care questions
- How has my caesarean birth shaped my feelings about birth and pregnancy?
- What actions can I take to support my own health and wellbeing and that of my baby (babies)?
- What is important to me in future family planning and future births?

What are the long-term outcomes of caesarean birth?

Before I begin to explore the long-term outcomes of caesarean birth, I want to explain that this chapter inevitably requires looking at the things that can go wrong. I encourage you to remember that decision-making about caesarean birth can be complex and it is important to consider the whole picture (including not only your individual clinical circumstances, but also your own preferences).

For you...

As we saw in Chapter 3, caesarean birth can result in several outcomes that have long-term consequences for women's health:

- An emergency hysterectomy (uncommon)[2]
- Bladder injury (rare)[3]
- Ureteric injury (rare)
- Death (very rare)[4]

Women who have had a previous caesarean birth (and indeed some other forms of gynaecological surgery) also have a higher chance of complications in future births, particularly an increased likelihood of developing:

Placental problems

In Chapter 3, we briefly discussed placenta praevia as a potential indication for caesarean birth. We will now discuss the ways in which the chances of this occurring increase with in subsequent pregnancies after caesarean birth.

Number of previous caesarean births	Chance of placenta praevia	Of those with placenta praevia, how many will have a morbidly adherent placenta?
1	0.6–1.3%	11–14%
2	1.1–2.3%	23–40%
3+	1.8–3.7	35–67%

The NICE caesarean guideline[5] notes that:

Morbidly adherent placenta is associated with serious maternal morbidity including major obstetric haemorrhage, transfusion of large quantities of blood products, hysterectomy and admission to an intensive care unit. However, [severe loss of blood] *and maternal death from morbidly adherent placenta is now rare in the UK (Cantwell R. et al., 2011). It is hoped that improved prenatal identification of such cases has contributed to this.*[6]

Uterine rupture

Uterine rupture is a rare, but potentially grave, complication of pregnancy and/or birth.[7] For women with an unscarred uterus, uterine rupture is rare (6.1/10,000 births, or 0.061%).[8] For women with a caesarean scar, it is uncommon. The RCOG Green Top Guideline for Birth After Caesarean recommends that: '*Women should be informed that planned VBAC is associated with an approximately 1 in 200 (0.5%) risk of uterine rupture.*'[9]

Making meaningful decisions about uterine rupture is complicated by the fact that we are not always all using the same definitions.[10] Nonetheless, it is important to be aware of the potential implications:[11]

- Uterine rupture is associated with a 6.2% perinatal death rate; *and*
- 14–33% of women who experience uterine rupture will require an emergency hysterectomy.

It is also important to consider your individual circumstances, as there is some evidence to suggest that different factors might increase or decrease your likelihood of experiencing a uterine rupture during your pregnancy or birth. Factors discussed in the RCOG Green Top Guideline include:

- *Onset of labour* (spontaneous labour has a lower likelihood of uterine rupture than induced or augmented labour).
- *Previous uterine rupture* (RCOG estimates that the chance of repeat uterine rupture in future births is at least 5%, and thus do not recommend planning a vaginal birth in these circumstances).
- *'Classical' caesarean scar* (a contraindication for planned VBAC, according to RCOG).
- *Previous vaginal delivery* (reduces the likelihood of uterine rupture).
- *Number of previous caesareans* (RCOG notes that the number of previous caesareans *does not* independently increase the likelihood of uterine rupture).
- *Other factors* associated with an increased likelihood or uterine rupture include:

- If it is less than 12 months since last birth
- Post-dates pregnancy
- Maternal age of 40 years or more
- Obesity
- Lower pre-labour Bishop score[12]
- Macrosomia (baby weighs more than 8lb 13oz)
- Concerns raised in ultrasound assessment of uterine thickness
- However, RCOG also note that: *'There is uncertainty in how to incorporate this knowledge in antenatal counselling and therefore the presence of these risk factors does not contraindicate VBAC.'* [13]

Stillbirth

Previous caesarean is one potential factor that has been associated with an increased likelihood of stillbirth (particularly stillbirth during labour itself).[14] This is partly connected to the complications described above (for example, the MMBRACE Perinatal Confidential Enquiry report, published in 2017, examined 14 perinatal deaths where the mother hah had a previous caesarean, and found that four related to uterine rupture).

The report notes that stillbirth is still an uncommon outcome of planned births after caesarean, but recommends that, in the antenatal period, there should be: 'Documentation of discussion and the agreed management plan for labour and birth following previous caesarean section'.

For your baby...

We don't really know. Yet... This is an unsatisfactory, but honest, assessment.

Below, I explore emerging evidence about associations between caesarean birth and various outcomes for babies and children.[15] Then I consider two widely debated, emerging areas of research with possible implications for caesarean birth (the microbiome and epigenetics).

NICE surveillance report 2017

The NICE Caesarean guideline doesn't include information on the relationship between caesarean birth and long-term outcomes. In 2017, NICE published a surveillance report of recent research,[16] which identified three systematic reviews that explored the longer-term impact of caesarean birth on babies:

- *Irritable Bowel Disease (IBD):* A systematic review of seven observational studies found that caesarean birth was not associated with a significant increase in the risk of IBD, including ulcerative colitis or Crohn's disease. NICE note a number of limitations of the studies, including not exploring different kinds of caesarean birth, nor different kinds of IBD.
- *Obesity:* A systematic review found an association between caesarean birth and increased BMI and an increased likelihood of being overweight and/or obese later in life, when compared to vaginal birth.

    NICE noted limitations in the study (notably that the studies included caesarean births from the 1990s, so may not reflect current practice, and that the impact of other factors remains unclear). They advise caution in the interpretation of these findings.
- *Asthma:* A systematic review of 26 cohort studies found an association between caesarean birth (and instrumental vaginal birth) and increased likelihood of asthma in children, compared to spontaneous vaginal birth. NICE noted several potential limitations, including an unclear risk of bias.

NICE is currently updating the Caesarean guideline to offer more up-to-date guidance on the long-term outcomes of caesarean birth. You can keep up-to-date by checking the NICE Caesarean guideline webpage. In the meantime, your caregivers should help you explore the advantages and disadvantages of caesarean birth in your circumstances.

The microbiome and caesarean birth

In 2014, filmmakers Toni Harman and Alex Wakeford released *Microbirth*, an award-winning documentary that explores 'the latest science about the 'seeding and feeding' of a baby's microbiome during pregnancy, birth and breastfeeding.'[17] This film, and their subsequent book, has prompted widespread discussion about the microbiome and its relevance to decision-making about caesarean birth. They write in *The Microbiome Effect*:

What is the microbiome?
The human microbiome comprises trillions of microorganisms that live on you and in you – the bacteria, fungi, viruses, protozoa and archea… These trillions of microbes play a very important role: they keep the body functioning and help protect you from disease.

How does this relate to childbirth?
The fetus develops in a near sterile environment in the womb, which means that childbirth is likely to be the baby's first contact with the world of microbes. During vaginal birth, as he or she travels through the birth canal, the baby is coated in the mother's bacteria. This payload of microbes goes straight into the baby's eyes and ears, up its nose, and into its mouth. Inevitably, the baby swallows some of them, too.
In the baby's gut the first bacteria to arrive start to colonise

and multiply. Special breastmilk sugars, called oligosaccharides, are indigestible to the baby, but they are there purely to feed the baby's newly seeded gut bacteria. This natural 'seed and feed' process is perfectly designed to set up the baby's gut microbiome in the optimal way.

As a c-section baby hasn't travelled all the way through the birth canal, the first microbes he or she comes into contact with (aside from possible prenatal exposure) are likely to come from a number of sources within the environment of the operating theatre, not from the mother's vaginal tract.

Why does this matter?
According to Dr Blaser's 'Missing Microbes' hypothesis the current plague of disease in industrialised nations could be related to the depletion of bacterial diversity in our gut microbiome. Antibiotics, modern diet and lifestyle, and an increase in the numbers of c-section births could all contribute to this reduced diversity.

Are there reasons to be cautious?
Yes. The authors of *The Microbiome Effect* stress that we need to think cautiously and critically about how we interpret the research findings. They absolutely need to be considered within the wider picture of your circumstances (clinical and personal), so that any decision you make can be the most appropriate one for you (and your baby).

In many ways, theories about the microbiome raise more questions than they do answers. Here are just a few examples:

- What happens if a woman's waters break before she has a caesarean birth?[18]
- What happens when babies are premature?
- How does this impact waterbirth?
- What happens to the microbiome after birth?[19]

Beyond birth... what can I do to support my baby's microbiome?

If you have already given birth by caesarean (or know that you will need to give birth this way), it can be hard to read about the potential impact of caesarean birth on your baby's microbiome and future health. We all want our babies to be as healthy as possible and might worry that our child's route to birth may have an irreversible impact.

I caught up with Toni Harman, co-creator of *Microbirth,* and asked her how parents can support the development of a healthy microbiome. She stressed that much of the research surrounding the microbiome is still very tentative, and new research may transform what we know. She also pointed out that birth is simply one step in a series of potentially significant steps in the development of a healthy immune system. Other things to consider include:

- Early skin-to-skin
- Exclusive breastfeeding
- A sensible approach to antibiotics (e.g. by asking 'Are there any alternative approaches to treating this?')
- Developing an understanding of pre- and probiotics
- Allowing a healthy amount of dirt into your children's lives
- Active lives
- A varied diet

What about vaginal seeding?

You may have heard women discussing, or seen news stories about, a potential new approach to artificially 'seeding' your baby's (or babies') microbiome after a caesarean birth. It is definitely a hot topic, with as many as 90% of obstetricians reporting that women have asked them about it.[20]

This approach is being researched by Dr Maria Gloria Dominguez Bello. A sterile swab (a bit like a tampon) is placed inside the mother's vagina before surgery, then removed and placed in a sterile dish until the baby is born, when the swab is wiped over the baby's mouth, face and body.

Vaginal seeding is controversial. Concerns centre around the currently unproven benefits and unknown risks. Dr Patrick O'Brien, from the RCOG, said:

> There is no robust evidence to suggest that vaginal seeding has any associated benefits. We would therefore not recommend it until more definitive research shows that it is not harmful and can in fact improve a child's digestive and/or immune system.[21]

However, as Positive Birth Movement founder Milli Hill reminds us:

> It's as if everyone's completely forgotten – perhaps in their scramble to portray mothers, yet again, as selfish feckless idiots – that babies actually come out of women's dirty, soggy, bacteria-laden vaginas every single day. That's what's supposed to happen folks![22]

What about epigenetics and caesarean birth?

Epigenetics is the study of biological mechanisms that turn genes on and off, and the research in this fascinating area of science is perhaps even more emerging than the science surrounding the microbiome.

For example, some studies have suggested a link between mode of delivery and epigenetic markers.[23] However, another recent study has suggested that there are no links.[24]

It's really hard to say too much more about epigenetics and caesarean birth at the moment, because there is a real likelihood that hypotheses and implications might change as we learn more and thus, it's hard for us to use this information to make informed choices.

What do I need to know about birth after caesarean?

'Once a caesarean, always a caesarean' wrote obstetrician Edwin Cragin in 1916. Was he right? Yes, if we consider his comments in the context in which he made them, as Uqwumadu notes:

> At that time, rickets and pelvic deformity were prevalent even in industrialised countries, syntocinon for augmentation of slow labour was unknown, and surgery was crude and dangerous. The primary Caesarean section was undertaken to save the life of an exhausted, dehydrated, ketotic, often pyrexial and delirious, moribund mother. [25]

And now? For the majority of women who have birthed by caesarean, a more accurate and modern update of this maxim would be 'once a caesarean, always a controversy'.[26]

As you begin exploring your birth choices after a caesarean birth, you will discover that there are lots of differing opinions about the best way to approach birth after caesarean.

Official recommendations about birth after caesarean

The RCOG Birth after Previous Caesarean Birth Green Top Guideline notes that:

> There is a consensus, endorsed by evidence-based systematic reviews and clinical guidelines, that planned VBAC is a safe and appropriate mode of delivery for the majority of pregnant women with a singleton previous lower segment caesarean delivery.

It goes on to note:

> Women who have had two or more prior lower segment caesarean deliveries may be offered VBAC after counselling by a senior obstetrician.

The NICE Caesarean guideline notes that:

Clinically there is little or no difference in the risk associated with a planned caesarean and a planned vaginal birth in women who have had up to 4 previous caesarean sections. If a woman chooses to plan a vaginal birth after she has previously given birth by caesarean section, she should be fully supported in her choice.

If I plan a vaginal birth, what do I need to know?

The 2017 National Maternity and Perinatal Audit found that across Britain, 41.9% of women plan a vaginal birth after caesarean (of whom 57.7% give birth vaginally).

Previous caesarean birth is listed in NICE guidelines as a previous complication that is associated with increased risks to you or your baby, and could be more effectively monitored or treated in an obstetric-led environment.

The RCOG Birth After Previous Caesarean Green Top Guideline states that:

Women should be advised to have continuous electronic foetal monitoring for the duration of planned VBAC, commencing at the onset of regular uterine contractions. (NB: this a Grade D recommendation – see RCOG's information about guidelines)

and:

Women should be advised that planned VBAC should be conducted in a suitably staffed and equipped delivery suite with continuous intrapartum care and monitoring with resources available for immediate caesarean delivery and advanced neonatal resuscitation. (NB: this is a good practice point, based on experience of the guideline development group)

It is important to note that these are recommendations about what is offered to you. There is no obligation upon you to accept obstetric-led care, a hospital birth or continuous monitoring.

We will explore the potential advantages and disadvantages of midwife-led care for women who are birthing after a caesarean below. For now though, let's take a more detailed look at what obstetric-led care might look like.

Both NICE and RCOG recommend that local NHS trusts develop care pathways for women who have had previous caesareans to allow for a detailed discussion of the benefits and risks of birth after caesarean. This need has been reinforced by the recent 2017 MMBRACE Perinatal Confidential Enquiry report.

As a result, care pathways will vary from hospital to hospital (and may also vary according to your clinical and personal circumstances). If previous caesarean is the only identified 'risk factor' in your pregnancy, you will likely see a midwife for most of your appointments and often these appointments can be held in your home, or in a local community venue, rather than in hospital. Your midwife will liaise closely with your named obstetrician throughout your pregnancy, discussing any concerns that arise and referring you for additional assessment as appropriate.[27]

Depending on your circumstances, your antenatal care may be very similar to your first pregnancy (although you may have fewer appointments overall as you have been pregnant before). However, there will be some differences.

Many trusts will have a specialist midwife (or a lead consultant) who will meet women at around 20 weeks to discuss how they felt about their previous birth (or births), as well as their plans for birth in their current pregnancy. Your counselling should include a personalised assessment of the risks and benefits of either a planned vaginal birth (VBAC, or VBA2C if you've had two previous caesareans) or repeat caesarean. You will also be offered another appointment with your midwife or obstetrician at around 36 weeks to finalise the plan for your birth.

If you plan a repeat caesarean, this will usually be booked in after 39 weeks. If you plan a vaginal birth, and do not go into labour by 40–41 weeks, you can expect to be invited to another appointment to plan the next steps in your care. Often this will be with an obstetrician, who can talk through the relative advantages and disadvantages of expectant management (waiting for spontaneous labour), induction (offering a sweep, or assessing if it would be possible to artificially 'break your waters') or booking a repeat caesarean.

Midwife-led care after caesarean

RCOG and NICE guidelines do not recommend midwife-led care during labour for women with a previous caesarean. Nonetheless, there is a significant minority of women who request midwife-led care (sometimes called 'out of guideline care').

In 2015, the NPEU published a follow-up report (as part of the wider Birthplace study). It found that although most 'higher risk' women planned to give birth in an obstetric-led setting, around 7% of women who planned home birth, 4% of those who planned birth in an co-located midwife-led unit, and 3% who planned birth in a freestanding midwife-led unit had known risk factors.

The NPEU report noted that:

The evidence on women's decision-making in planning birth at home suggests that they are motivated by the desire to avoid the perceived 'risks' of intervention associated with birth in an [obstetric unit], in part because of previous negative experiences, as well as valuing greater control and wanting a relaxing and comfortable environment.

They also noted that 'higher risk' women who planned birth at home or in a freestanding unit were more likely to already have children and to be older, white, married or living with a partner and living in less deprived areas than 'higher risk' women who planned obstetric unit birth. By contrast 'higher risk' women who planned birth in a co-located unit were more similar to the obstetric unit group.

'Higher risk' women planning births in an obstetric unit tended to have different clinical circumstances to 'higher risk' women planning a birth in a midwife-led setting (i.e. they had different 'risk' factors and were more likely to have more than one 'risk' factor). Previous caesarean and 'post-dates' pregnancy were common in both obstetric and non-obstetric settings, but women with pre-eclampsia, for example, tended to plan a birth in an obstetric setting.

On average, the transfer rate was around 50% for first time 'higher risk' pregnancies and 20% for subsequent 'higher risk' pregnancies.

The study found that the likelihood of adverse outcomes was higher for 'higher risk' women who planned to give birth in midwife-led settings than it was for women who were considered to be 'low risk'.

A couple of things to note:

- Sample size limitations make it difficult to explore individual risk factors (so we can't know how this affects previous caesarean as a risk factor); and
- Neither the Birthplace study (nor the other studies they cite) compare with 'higher risk' women who plan births in an obstetric unit.

What do I need to know if I plan a repeat caesarean?

We have already covered many aspects of planning a caesarean birth. Nonetheless, a few points bear reiteration here:

- *Family planning expectations.* We saw in the previous section that the chances of experiencing complications increase with the number of caesareans that you have.
- *The importance of planning a caesarean after 39 weeks* (unless there is a clinical need to expedite your birth). This has been shown to reduce the likelihood of respiratory complications after birth.
- *The possibility that you might go into labour before your planned caesarean date.* This happens quite often and it is a great idea to talk through what will happen if you go into labour unexpectedly, particularly if this happens at night.

Conclusion

What I hope has become clear throughout this book is that caesarean birth matters primarily because you matter.

Decision-making about caesarean birth is not always easy. I hope that this book will support you to have meaningful discussions with your caregivers about the options available to you so that you can feel confident in your decisions. There is more than one 'right' way.

Caesarean birth can be an amazing experience. I hope that the words I have written here will help you feel prepared for birth in theatre, and inspired to personalise your experience. There is no 'one size fits all'.

Caesarean recovery is different for everyone. I hope this book helps you find the support you need as you recover and grow into your new role as a mother. You matter just as much as your new baby (or babies)!

Finally, I hope this book draws out your voice. Let's work together to put women at the centre of caesarean birth.

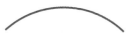

References

Introduction
1   Rebecca Solnit 'Silence and Powerlessness Go Hand in Hand: Women's Voices Must Be Heard' in the Guardian.
2   I use Positive Birth Movement founder Milli Hill's definition: 'A positive birth means a birth in which a woman feels she has freedom of choice, access to accurate information, and that she is in control, powerful and respected.'

Chapter 1
1   A significant minority of women choose to birth without a healthcare professional in attendance ('freebirth'), or completely alone. See Feeley and Thompson's 'Why do some women choose to freebirth in the UK? An interpretative phenomenological study'.
2   Vanessa Olorenshaw, *Liberating Motherhood: Birthing the Purplestockings Movement*, Womancraft, 2016, p10.
3   Taken from NHS Maternity Statistics 2016-17.
4   Taken from the Select Committee on Health Fourth Report (Session 2002-3).
5   I have seen many different data sources and definitions of a caesarean rate. Here I refer to the Maternity Services Monthly Statistics, England, April 2018, experimental statistics.
6   For a definition of high-risk, see Tables 39-42 in the full NICE Guideline 190 for Intrapartum Care, p37-39 (version updated in May 2017).
7   www.theguardian.com/commentisfree/2016/dec/07/caesarean-sec-

tions-mother-blaming-small-pelvises

8   www.who.int/reproductivehealth/publications/maternal_perinatal_health/
    cs-statement/en/. The WHO's most recent statement softens its stance on the
    'ideal' caesarean rate: 'At population level, caesarean section rates higher than
    10% are not associated with reductions in maternal and newborn mortality
    rates'. The WHO used to say 'there is no justification for any region to have
    a rate higher than 10-15%'. This statement was criticised for not being based
    on strong evidence.

9   jamanetwork.com/journals/jama/fullarticle/2473490

10 The RCOG guidance for Presenting Information on Risk notes that anything
    from 1/100 to 1/1,000 is 'uncommon'. The Birthplace study notes: 'For 'low
    risk' women the incidence of adverse perinatal outcomes…was low (4.3
    events per 1,000 births)'.

11 '[The UK's] maternal mortality rate [of less than 1/10,000] is lower than
    age-matched male death rates (5-17 per 10,000 for men aged 20-44 years in
    England and Wales). *Lancet*, 2017.

12 2015 World Bank data shows that the neonatal mortality rate was 28/1,000
    (2.8%) and the maternal mortality rate was 475/100,000 (0.475%). But mor-
    tality is not the only adverse outcome, nor should we place too much weight
    on data that may have limitations.

13 Each Baby Counts: 2015

14 More about absolute indications for caesarean birth: www.ncbi.nlm.nih.gov/
    pmc/articles/PMC4555060/

15 A.U. Lokugamage, 'Human rights in childbirth, narratives and restorative
    justice – a review'.

16 RCOG consent guidelines say: '[caesarean birth is appropriate] to secure the
    safest and/or quickest route of delivery in the circumstances present at the
    time the decision is made, where the anticipated risks to mother and/or baby
    of an alternative mode of delivery outweigh those of caesarean section'.

17 matexp.org.uk/matexp-and-me/in-the-shoes-of-florence-wilcock-division-
    al-director-specialist-services-obstetrician-kingston-hospital-ft/

18 A.U. Lokugamage, 'Human rights in childbirth, narratives and restorative
    justice – a review'.

19 It can be difficult for health care professionals to offer this in the current
    maternity system, and I am not assigning blame, rather calling on all of us to
    tackle this together.

20 The WHO includes a helpful infographic explaining the Robson Groups on
    p6 of their statement on Caesarean Section Rates.

21 World Health Report 2010, Background paper 30 by Luz Gibbons et al.

22 Betran, A.P. (et al) 'Rates of caesarean section: analysis of global, regional
    and national estimates'.

23 From WHO information about Millennium Development Goal 5: www.
    who.int/topics/millennium_development_goals/maternal_health/en/

24 From WHO World Health Statistics 2015 Report: www.who.int/reproduc-
    tivehealth/topics/mdgs/health-service-coverage2015.pdf
25 From WHO Global Health Observatory Data repository: apps.who.int/gho/
    data/view.main.1370?lang=en
26 From WHO World Health Statistics 2015 Report: www.who.int/reproduc-
    tivehealth/topics/mdgs/health-service-coverage2015.pdf
27 *BMJ* Research News: www.bmj.com/content/350/bmj.h1332
28 For further discussion: www.acog.org/Resources-And-Publications/Com-
    mittee-Opinions/Committee-on-Health-Care-for-Underserved-Women/
    Health-Care-Systems-for-Underserved-Women#10
29 For example: www.plannedparenthoodaction.org/blog/how-the-trump-ad-
    ministration-has-threatened-womens-health-in-just-a-few-months
30 'Caesarean Section in the World: a new ecological approach': www.ncbi.nlm.
    nih.gov/pubmed/22442920
31 'Cesarean section rates and maternal and neonatal mortality in low-, medi-
    um-, and high-income countries: an ecological study': www.ncbi.nlm.nih.
    gov/pubmed/17150064
32 reports.weforum.org/global-gender-gap-report-2016/top-ten/
33 A.U. Lokugamage, 'Human rights in childbirth, narratives and restorative
    justice – a review.'

Chapter 2
1 A.U. Lokugamage, 'Human rights in childbirth, narratives and restorative
   justice – a review'. Also note that this idea is not from the very distant past.
2 Rebecca Schiller, *Why Human Rights in Childbirth Matter*, p136
3 Rebecca Schiller, *Why Human Rights in Childbirth Matter*, p136
4 In rare cases a woman may lack 'mental capacity' to make decisions, but
   this does not negate the emphasis that: 'A mentally competent woman may
   refuse treatment even where it might cause death or serious harm to her or
   her baby' (Schiller, 2016).
5 Trisha Greenhalgh, 'Evidence Based Medicine: a Movement in Crisis?' *BMJ*.
6 One 2005 24-hour audit of an acute hospital included 18 patients with 44
   diagnoses; 3,679 pages of national guidelines (122 hours of reading) were
   relevant to their immediate care. Trisha Greenhalgh: www.bmj.com/con-
   tent/348/bmj.g3725
7 Greenhalgh writes: 'evidence based medicine has drifted in recent years
   from investigating and managing established disease to detecting and inter-
   vening in non-diseases. Risk assessment using 'evidence based' scores and al-
   gorithms (for heart disease, diabetes, cancer, and osteoporosis, for example)
   now occurs on an industrial scale, with scant attention to the opportunity
   costs or unintended human and financial consequences'.
8 www.kingsfund.org.uk/sites/files/kf/field/field_publication_file/pa-
   tients-preferences-matter-may-2012.pdf

9 www.england.nhs.uk/wp-content/uploads/2016/02/national-maternity-re-view-report.pdf

10 Jean Walker 'Informed Choice and the Concept of Risk', RCM.

11 www.kingsfund.org.uk/sites/files/kf/field/field_publication_file/pa-tients-preferences-matter-may-2012.pdf

12 Jean Walker 'Informed Choice and the Concept of Risk', RCM.

13 Milli Hill, The Positive Birth Book, p73

14 Lucy Pearce, Burning Woman p8

15 Milli Hill The Positive Birth Book, p154

16 Brené Brown 'Why your critics aren't the ones who count'. www.youtube.com/watch?v=8-JXOnFOXQk&feature=youtu.be

Chapter 3

1 Courtney Key Jarecki. Homebirth Cesarean, p47

2 Magnus Murphy and Pauline McDonagh Hull, Choosing Cesarean- a Natu-ral Birth Plan, p29

3 Ideally these conversations happen antenatally or as circumstances change, but sometimes there isn't time. If that is the case, meaningful conversations must happen afterwards.

4 Homebirth Cesarean, p50

5 Homebirth Cesarean, p73

6 If you live outside the UK, see Chapter 1. In Scotland, the provisional cae-sarean birth rate for 2016 was 32.4% (15% elective and 17.4% emergency). In Wales, the caesarean birth rate in 2014-15 was 26.4% (11.3% elective and 15.1% emergency). In Northern Ireland, caesarean section birth rates (at just over 28 per cent) were broadly in line with the national average.

7 The Birthplace study found that for healthy women giving birth in obstetric led environments, on average 11% give birth by caesarean, which is still much lower than the overall national average.

8 The data from the Sentinel Audit is 17 years out of date but is still some of the most comprehensive data that we have. Use the data with an open mind, acknowledging that the caesarean rate has risen significantly since 2001.

9 As noted in the National Sentinel Caesarean Section Audit, p3.

10 Mylonas et al 'Indications for and risks of elective caesarean section'.

11 RCOG, 'Patterns of Maternity Care in English NHS Trusts 2013/4'.

12 NICE grading system: www.ncbi.nlm.nih.gov/pubmedhealth/PMH0078457/ Most organisations creating evidence-based guidelines follow this system.

13 NICE Caesarean Guideline, p70.

14 'RCOG and Oxford Breech Conferences, October 2014' at: www.breechbirth.org.uk

15 www.ncbi.nlm.nih.gov/pubmed/28029180/

16 www.nice.org.uk/guidance/cg132

17 Hands Off that Breech www.aims.org.uk and the RCOG patient leaflet www.rcog.org.uk/en/patients/patient-leaflets/breech-baby-at-the-end-of-pregnancy/

18 www.obstetrics-gynaecology-journal.com/article/S1751-7214(07)00142-X/abstract

19 NICE Caesarean guideline, p73. Caesarean rates vary by gestational age: at term 60% women with a twin pregnancy had a CS, while at less than 28 weeks the caesarean rate was less than 29%. Where caesarean was planned for multiple pregnancy, breech presentation of the first twin was the most commonly reported indication (14%), together with previous caesarean (7%), and maternal request (9%). Of the unplanned caesarean sections, fetal distress was the most influential factor in 29% and 'failure to progress' in 12%. Almost all triplet pregnancies (92%) were delivered by caesarean.

20 www.nice.org.uk/donotdo/the-risk-of-neonatal-morbidity-and-mortality-is-higher-with-small-for-gestationalage-babies-however-the-effect-of-planned-caesarian-section-cs-in-improving-these-outcomes-remains-uncertain-and

21 www.nice.org.uk/guidance/cg190/evidence/full-guideline-pdf-248734770

22 RCOG patient information leaflet: www.rcog.org.uk/globalassets/documents/patients/patient-information-leaflets/pregnancy/umbilical-cord-prolapse-in-late-pregnancy.pdf

23 RCOG Green Top Guideline for Umbilical Cord Prolapse, p5.

24 www.rcog.org.uk/globalassets/documents/guidelines/goodpractice11classificationofurgency.pdf

25 RCOG Green Top Guideline for Umbilical Cord Prolapse.

26 NICE Caesarean guideline, p76-7

27 www.npeu.ox.ac.uk/downloads/files/mbrrace-uk/reports/MBRRACE-UK%20Maternal%20Report%202016%20-%20website.pdf

28 www.rcog.org.uk/globalassets/documents/guidelines/gtg_63.pdf

29 www.rcog.org.uk/globalassets/documents/patients/patient-information-leaflets/pregnancy/heavy-bleeding-after-birth.pdf

30 Also referred to as 'failure to progress'; I have not used that term because it is negative and can feel shaming.

31 The NICE Intrapartum Care guideline provides information about diagnosing delay in labour in the first (dilation from 4-10cm) and second (pushing stage) stages of labour.

32 Note that NICE guidelines state that: 'Pelvimetry is not useful in predicting 'failure to progress' in labour and should not be used in decision making about mode of birth' and 'Shoe size, maternal height and estimations of fetal size (ultrasound or clinical examination) do not accurately predict cephalopelvic disproportion and should not be used to predict 'failure to progress' during labour.'

33 www.nhs.uk/conditions/pregnancy-and-baby/pages/pregnancy-infections.aspx

34 The Birthplace study follow-up report notes that: 'recent research using the

Birthplace data suggests that otherwise healthy multiparous women with a BMI of 35– 40 kg/m2 may have relatively low intrapartum risks, and a Dutch study found that extremely obese women achieved good outcomes in midwifery-led care.'

35 'Uterine rupture is still rare among women who have had a previous caesarean section and plan to have a normal birth at 21 per 10,000 pregnancies. But this is higher than in those who elect for another caesarean section, where the incidence is 3 per 10,000 births.' www.npeu.ox.ac.uk/ukoss/news/31-uterine-rupture-is-rarer-than-previously-thought

36 The NHS Litigation Authority identified 85 claims relating to uterine rupture between 2000-10, valued at over £100m.

37 www.npeu.ox.ac.uk/ukoss/current-surveillance/ur

38 www.networks.nhs.uk/nhs-networks/staffordshire-shrop-shire-and-black-country/documents/Uterine%20Rupture%202013.pdf and www.royalberkshire.nhs.uk/Downloads/GPs/GP%20protocols%20and%20 guidelines/Maternity%20Guidelines%20and%20Policies/Intrapartum/Rup-tured%20Uterus_V5.0_GL908.pdf

39 www.nice.org.uk/guidance/cg107

40 www.ncbi.nlm.nih.gov/pmc/articles/PMC3008318/

41 Tita and Andrews 'Diagnosis and Management of Clinical Chorioamnionitis'.

Chapter 4

1 Not all opinions are of equal benefit to you. An obstetrician will likely have more evidence-based information than an average person, but a lay person who really values you and what you want may be better suited to helping you weigh up the evidence than a time-pressed healthcare professional.

2 www.nice.org.uk/guidance/cg132/chapter/appendix-c-planned-cs-com-pared-with-planned-vaginal-birth

3 Evidence was identified about caesarean and its impact on maternal outcomes (risk of future ectopic pregnancy, stillbirth or miscarriage, sub-fertility) and infant outcomes (cerebral palsy, childhood obesity, asthma, bowel disease, and iron-related haematological indices).

4 www.rcog.org.uk/en/guidelines-research-services/guidelines/consent-advice-7/

5 www.nhs.uk/Conditions/Respiratory-distress-syndrome/Pages/Introduction.aspx

6 www.nhs.uk/Conditions/pulmonary-hypertension/Pages/causes.aspx

7 Iatrogenic prematurity refers to the birth of a physiologically immature and/or low-weight infant who is delivered prematurely as a result of medical intervention. Sometimes this is necessary, other times it is accidental, which is why elective caesarean are usually planned for after 39 weeks.

8 Reported in the RCOG's 'Patterns of maternity care in English NHS Trusts 2013-4'.

9   See their Clinical Report 2017.
10 www.rcog.org.uk/en/guidelines-research-services/guidelines/consent-advice-11/
11 www.rcm.org.uk/news-views-and-analysis/analysis/how-to-perform-an-episiotomy and www.rcog.org.uk/globalassets/documents/guidelines/gtg-29.pdf
12 www.rcog.org.uk/en/patients/patient-leaflets/third--or-fourth-degree-tear-during-childbirth/
13 www.rcog.org.uk/globalassets/documents/patients/patient-information-leaflets/pregnancy/pi-shoulder-dystocia.pdf
14 www.rcog.org.uk/globalassets/documents/patients/patient-information-leaflets/gynaecology/pi-pelvic-organ-prolapse.pdf
15 From: www.rcog.org.uk/globalassets/documents/patients/patient-information-leaflets/pregnancy/heavy-bleeding-after-birth.pdf

Chapter 5
1   Quotes from: www.positivebirthmovement.org/pbm-blog/reflecting-on-experiences-around-risk-during-pregnancy-and-birth
2   Recommendations about place of birth have been removed from the caesarean guideline, because they were addressed in the NICE Intrapartum Care guideline.
3   www.cochrane.org/CD004945/PREG_induction-of-labour-in-women-with-normal-pregnancies-at-or-beyond-term
4   apps.who.int/iris/bitstream/10665/44145/4/9789241546669_4_eng.pdf
5   According to the NICE Caesarean guideline: 'In maternity units where consultant obstetricians were frequently involved either in the decision for CS or present in theatre for 'emergency' CS the crude and adjusted CS rates (having taken into account case mix differences) were lower.'
6   stratog.rcog.org.uk/tutorial/obstetrics/fetal-blood-sampling-5811
7   www.npeu.ox.ac.uk/birthplace
8   In the obstetric unit, 80.5% had no complicating conditions at the start of labour, compared to 93.1% for homebirths. Complicating factors include: premature rupture of membranes (18+ hours), meconium stained liquor, proteinuria, hypertension, abnormal vaginal bleeding, non-cephalic presentation and abnormal heart rate.
9   Some women in obstetric units may be transferred during labour to units with greater capacity for high-dependency care. These numbers are very low: 1% in first pregnancies and 0.4% subsequently.
10 Defined as: stillbirth during labour, death of the baby in the first week after birth, neonatal encephalopathy, meconium aspiration syndrome, physical birth injuries such as brachial plexus injury and bone fractures.
11 Milli Hill, *The Positive Birth Book*, p187.
12 From: cambridgevbacfriends.wordpress.com/2015/11/11/ra-

chels-home-vbac-gentle-caesarean-birth

13 www.rcog.org.uk/globalassets/documents/guidelines/consent-advice/ca7-15072010.pdf

14 From RCM's Evidence Based Guidelines for Supporting Women in Labour.

15 From Sheila Kitzinger Symposium summary report 'Relationships, the pathway to safe, high quality maternity care', p7.

16 Taken from the CQC's Statistical release for the 2017 survey of women's experiences of maternity care, p3.

17 Full report: www.nct.org.uk/sites/default/files/related_documents/Support_Overdue_2017.pdf

18 www.rcm.org.uk/sites/default/files/Complementary%20Therapies%20and%20Natural%20Remedies_3.pdf

Chapter 6

1 southwarkbelle.blogspot.co.uk/search?updat-ed-max=2016-03-24T20:28:00Z&max-results=7)

2 www.the-pool.com/life/parenting-honestly/2017/23/up-with-the-kids-robyn-wilder-on-defending-right-to-a-caesarean

3 www.rcog.org.uk/en/patients/patient-leaflets/induction-of-labour---infor-mation-for-people-who-use-nhs-services/

4 apps.who.int/iris/bitstream/10665/44121/1/9789241547734_eng.pdf

5 The same accountability needs to be applied to midwives, who have a huge impact on the likelihood of caesarean, so it should be a joint review.

6 At its simplest, commissioning is the process of planning, agreeing and monitoring services. However, securing services is more complicated than securing goods and the intricacy of NHS services is unparalleled. www.england.nhs.uk/commissioning/

7 www.nice.org.uk/guidance/cg132/resources/costing-report-184766797

8 www.supremecourt.uk/decided-cases/docs/UKSC_2013_0136_Judgment.pdf

9 www.birthrights.org.uk/2017/05/do-i-have-a-right-to-choose-a-caesarean-section/

Chapter 7

1 @DerbyBOTB on Twitter. One staff member noted: 'it demonstrated how disempowering and emotional going to theatre can be (and we were not frightened or in pain)'.

2 Vaginal birth varies too: it can be physiological or assisted, frightening or empowering and quick or slow.

3 www.rcog.org.uk/globalassets/documents/guidelines/goodpractice11classi-ficationofurgency.pdf

4 These are: placental abruption, cord prolapse, uterine rupture, actively bleed-ing placenta praevia, intrapartum haemorrhage, presumed fetal compromise

with severely abnormal CTG or an FBS pH less than 7.2. Of the 16% of cases reported to be in category 1, 51% filled these criteria. 2001 National Sentinel Caesarean Section Audit.

5   NICE Caesarean guideline.
6   www.oaa-anaes.ac.uk/ui/content/content.aspx?id=175
7   ghostwritermummy.co.uk/2016/04/16/what-happens-when-you-dont-listen-to-women/
8   RCOG Caesarean Consent guidelines
9   www.nice.org.uk/guidance/cg132/evidence/full-guideline-pdf-184810861 p135
10 www.nice.org.uk/guidance/CG74/chapter/1-Guidance see 1.2.2 and 1.2.3
11 Adapted from Florence Wilcock's blog: matexp.org.uk/category/caesarean-sections/
12 Learn more here: www.laleche.org.uk/antenatal-expression-of-colostrum/#pregnant and www.nhs.uk/Conditions/pregnancy-and-baby/Pages/expressing-storing-breast-milk.aspx#hand
13 www.nrls.npsa.nhs.uk/resources/clinical-specialty/pregnancy-and-birth/?entryid45=83972
14 matexp.org.uk/the-matexp-journey/caesarean-sections/
15 For example, www.scarymommy.com/what-is-gentle-c-section/
16 www.ncbi.nlm.nih.gov/pmc/articles/PMC2613254/
17 Milli Hill, *The Positive Birth Book*
18 betterbirths.rcm.org.uk/baby-friendly-caesarean-section/
19 A Cochrane Review looked at the impact of music during caesarean birth, concluding: 'music during planned caesarean section under regional anaesthesia may improve pulse rate and birth satisfaction score. However, the magnitude of these benefits is small and the methodological quality of the one included trial is questionable. Therefore, the clinical significance of music is unclear'.
20 For discussion: www.optimumdoula.co.uk/cordties.html
21 This process is described in detail in: www.ncbi.nlm.nih.gov/pmc/articles/PMC2613254/
22 matexp.org.uk/category/caesarean-sections/
23 Full story here: www.positivebirthmovement.org/birth-story-a-healing-general-anaesthetic-caesarean/
24 www.nice.org.uk/guidance/cg132/evidence/full-guideline-pdf-184810861 p175.
25 onlinelibrary.wiley.com/doi/10.1002/14651858.CD011216/full
26 www.ncbi.nlm.nih.gov/pubmed/18818022
27 For a positive story: www.positivebirthmovement.org/pbm-blog/birth-story-a-healing-general-anaesthetic-caesarean
28 Taken from www.labourpains.com
29 www.pinterandmartin.com/why-mothers-medication-matters.html

30 www.cochrane.org/CD011216/complementary-and-alternative-thera-pies-post-caesarean-pain

31 www.closingthebonesmassage.com

32 www.unicef.org.uk/babyfriendly/baby-friendly-resources/imple   ment-ing-standards-resources/skin-to-skin-contact/

33 www.cochrane.org/CD003519/PREG_early-skin-skin-contact-mothers-and-their-healthy-newborn-infants

34 www.unicef.org.uk/babyfriendly/baby-friendly-resources/guid-ance-for-health-professionals/implementing-the-baby-friendly-standards/further-guidance-on-implementing-the-standards/skin-to-skin-contact/ and www.unicef.org.uk/babyfriendly/news-and-research/baby-friendly-re-search/research-supporting-breastfeeding/skin-to-skin-contact/

35 NICE did not identify any studies addressing the specific thermal require-ment of babies born by caesarean and recommended further research.

36 A systematic review published on the Cochrane database noted: 'Women practicing [skin-to-skin contact – SSC] after cesarean birth were probably more likely to breast feed one to four months post birth and to breast feed successfully (IBFAT score), but analyses were based on just two trials and few women. Evidence was insufficient to determine whether SSC could improve breastfeeding at other times after cesarean. Single trials contributed to infant respiratory rate, maternal pain and maternal state anxiety with no power to detect group differences'.

37 NICE Caesarean guideline, p164

38 As seen in research studies like this: bmcpregnancychildbirth.biomedcen-tral.com/articles/10.1186/1471-2393-10-21

39 www.positivebirthmovement.org/birth-story-a-healing-general-anaesthet-ic-caesarean/

40 A survey of policy at 1,175 units in 14 European countries found that two-thirds clamped the cord immediately after birth. www.rcog.org.uk/globalas-sets/documents/guidelines/scientific-impact-papers/sip-14.pdf

41 onlinelibrary.wiley.com/doi/10.1002/14651858.CD004074.pub3/full

42 www.nhs.uk/conditions/jaundice-newborn/treatment/

43 www.who.int/elena/titles/full_recommendations/cord_clamping/en/

44 www.nice.org.uk/guidance/qs105/chapter/quality-statement-6-de-layed-cord-clamping

45 According to NICE expert opinion: 'Concerns would arise over cord integ-rity if the cord was damaged in any way, if it had snapped during delivery or if there was bleeding to the cord. Definitions of cord integrity are not limited to those stated here.'

46 According to NICE: 'Concern would arise if, after delivery, the baby has a heartbeat below 60 beats/minute that is not getting faster.'

47 www.who.int/elena/titles/full_recommendations/cord_clamping/en/

48 www.rcog.org.uk/globalassets/documents/guidelines/scientific-impact-pa-

pers/sip-14.pdf
49 www.cochrane.org/CD007555/PREG_alternative-positions-for-the-ba-
    by-immediately-at-birth-before-clamping-the-umbilical-cord
50 www.fatherhoodinstitute.org/2014/fi-research-summary-fathers-at-the-
    birth/
51 NSPCC's All Babies Count Dads' project: www.nspcc.org.uk/ser-
    vices-and-resources/research-and-resources/2014/all-babies-count-dad-
    project/
52 Mark Harris, *Men, Love & Birth*, p21
53 Partners are not always entitled to time off for antenatal appointments and
    education (unlike pregnant women).

Chapter 8
1   ghostwritermummy.co.uk/2016/04/12/pain-after-a-c-section/
2   The NICE CG132 guideline notes that the following should be recorded:
    level of consciousness, haemoglobin saturation and oxygen administration,
    blood pressure, respiratory frequency, heart rate and rhythm, pain intensity,
    intravenous infusions and drugs administered.
3   Women who have caesareans due to uterine rupture, maternal medical
    conditions and actively bleeding placenta praevia tend to be most likely to be
    admitted to ICU. NICE caesarean guideline, p166.
4   www.bliss.org.uk/statistics-about-neonatal-care and www.nhs.uk/Condi-
    tions/pregnancy-and-baby/pages/baby-special-intensive-care.aspx
5   A systematic review found no evidence to justify the restriction of food and
    drink after an uncomplicated caesarean. www.cochrane.org/CD003516/
    PREG_early-compared-with-delayed-oral-fluids-and-food-after-caesarean-
    section
6   www.cochrane.org/CD011562/PREG_does-chewing-gum-after-caesare-
    an-section-lead-quicker-recovery-bowel-function
7   www.nhs.uk/Conditions/pregnancy-and-baby/Pages/newborn-screening.
    aspx
8   www.uhs.nhs.uk/Media/Controlleddocuments/Patientinformation/Preg-
    nancyandbirth/Enhancedrecoveryfromelectivecaesareansection-patientin-
    formation.pdf
9   More information here: www.bwnft.nhs.uk/wp-content/uploads/2012/06/
    images_downloads_pdf_159_postn_clexane.pdf
10 NICE Caesarean Guideline, p9.
11 When to seek medical advice: www.nhs.uk/conditions/caesarean-section/
    recovery/ and postnatal depression: www.nhs.uk/Conditions/pregnan-
    cy-and-baby/Pages/feeling-depressed-after-birth.aspx
12 Read more here: www.huffingtonpost.com/damon-young/men-just-dont-
    trust-women_b_6714280.html?guccounter=1
13 Courtney Key Jarecki, *Homebirth Cesarean* p163.

14 Vanessa Olorenshaw, *Liberating Motherhood*, p156

15 www.psychologytoday.com/basics/attachment

16 Sutton Trust research highlights that insecure attachment is associated with poverty, mental health challenges, young parenting, disabilities and low-quality early childcare.

17 NHS 'Bonding after Birth', from: www.nhs.uk/news/pregnancy-and-child/bonding-after-birth/

18 Breastfeeding challenges are common and not limited to women who birth by caesarean. The 2010 Infant Feeding Survey showed that the prevalence of breastfeeding fell from 81% at birth to 69% at one week and 55% at six weeks.

19 NICE Caesarean guideline p164

20 In the non-intention to treat analysis (i.e. when looking at actual mode of birth, rather than planned mode of birth), 73–77% of women who had a vaginal birth and 65–67% of those who had caesarean, had breastfed at three months after birth.

21 In a UK-based population study (of 202 women) 'breastfeeding rates were 76% among those who delivered vaginally and 39% among those who had a CS'.

22 NICE Caesarean guideline p164

23 en.oxforddictionaries.com/definition/give_birth

24 Lucy Pearce, *Burning Woman*, p196

25 strongsincebirth.wordpress.com/tag/informed-choice/

26 Vanessa Olorenshaw, *Liberating Motherhood*, p63

27 Courtney Key Jarecki, *Homebirth Cesarean*, p35

28 Magnus Murphy and Pauline McDonagh Hull, *Choosing Cesarean: a Natural Birth Plan*, p33

29 strongsincebirth.wordpress.com

30 Lucy Pearce, *Burning Woman*, p196

31 birthwithoutfearblog.com/2015/09/14/i-am-strong-because-i-am-free/

32 birthwithoutfearblog.com/2015/12/15/i-am-strong-emily-weber/

33 Milli Hill, *The Positive Birth Book*, p287

34 Evidence base surrounding the benefits and harms of debriefing birth is still emerging. NICE notes: 'More RCT evidence is required to determine the effect of midwifery-led debriefing following CS.' See also: www.cochrane.org/CD007194/DEPRESSN_debriefing-interventions-for-the-prevention-of-psychological-trauma-in-women-following-childbirth, www.cochrane.org/CD000560/DEPRESSN_psychological-debriefing-for-preventing-post-traumatic-stress-disorder-ptsd and www.rcm.org.uk/learning-and-career/learning-and-research/ebm-articles/what-is-the-purpose-of-debriefing-women-in

35 NICE Caesarean guideline.

36 'Czarnocka and Slade (2000) have demonstrated that over 25% of women

following birth showed significant symptoms of psychological trauma, with Ayers (2004) concluding that one-third of women consider their experience of childbirth as traumatic.' www.rcm.org.uk/learning-and-career/learning-and-research/ebm-articles/exploring-women's-experiences-of-a-birth

37 '2% to 7% of women will experience PTSD at six weeks postnatally. Psychological debriefing was initially considered good practice to reduce the symptoms of PTSD, but is now a controversial intervention (Ayers, 2006)' From: www.rcm.org.uk/learning-and-career/learning-and-research/ebm-articles/exploring-women's-experiences-of-a-birth

Chapter 9

1 www.bbc.co.uk/news/science-environment-38210837

2 More about hysterectomy: www.nhs.uk/conditions/hysterectomy/ and www.hysterectomy-association.org.uk

3 For further discussion www.ncbi.nlm.nih.gov/pmc/articles/PMC4033551/

4 More about maternal and perinatal deaths: www.npeu.ox.ac.uk/mbrrace-uk

5 NICE Caesarean guideline, p77.

6 More about the guidelines for this care here: www.nrls.npsa.nhs.uk/resources/?EntryId45=66359

7 This video describes a 'true' or catastrophic uterine rupture: www.youtube.com/watch?v=3NOVCpIDWdE

8 patient.info/doctor/uterine-rupture

9 They explain that: 'The US Agency for Healthcare Research and Quality (AHRQ) meta-analysis and studies from the UK, Australia and Ireland reported a VBAC uterine rupture risk of 0.5%, 0.2%, 0.33% and 0.2% respectively. Rates of uterine rupture differ according to whether VBAC labour is spontaneous (0.15–0.4%), induced (0.54–1.4%) or augmented (0.9–1.91%). In the UK cohort study, two women with uterine rupture died (uterine rupture case fatality 1.3%, 95% CI 0.2–4.5%).'

10 www.bmj.com/rapid-response/2011/10/29/what-definition-uterine-rupture and midwifethinking.com/2016/06/15/vbac-making-a-mountain-out-of-a-molehill/

11 From an Evidence Report prepared for the Agency for Healthcare Research and Quality: www.ahrq.gov/downloads/pub/evidence/pdf/vbacup/vbacup.pdf

12 en.wikipedia.org/wiki/Bishop_score

13 RCOG Birth after Previous Caesarean Green Top Guideline, p8

14 The MMBRACE UK Perinatal Confidential Enquiry report (2017), found that: 'Studies have highlighted factors which are associated with intrapartum-related perinatal death, although most of the data has focused on intrapartum stillbirth. These factors can be grouped into maternal and fetal conditions... Maternal demographic characteristics and medical conditions include cigarette smoking, maternal age >35, prior caesarean section,

diabetes and hypertensive disorders. Fetal conditions include a small for gestational age baby and infection.'

15 www.nice.org.uk/guidance/cg132/evidence/appendix-a-summary-of-new-evidence-pdf-2736386032 and www.nice.org.uk/guidance/cg132/resources/surveillance-report-2017-caesarean-section-2011-nice-guideline-cg132-2736386033/chapter/Commentary-on-selected-new-evidence?tab=evidence.

16 www.nice.org.uk/guidance/cg132/resources/surveillance-report-2017-caesarean-section-2011-nice-guideline-cg132-2736386033/chapter/Surveillance-decision?tab=evidence

17 microbirth.com

18 One study noted: 'It stands to reason that a fetus delivered after arrest at 8 centimeters dilation after a long labor would be exposed to a much different microbial environment than a fetus that undergoes [caesarean delivery] for maternal request prior to rupture of membranes'. www.ncbi.nlm.nih.gov/pmc/articles/PMC3110651/

19 A 2017 study found that 'among infants 6 weeks of age, [there was] no substantial difference in microbiome diversity or pattern among those born via vaginal or cesarean delivery'. www.medscape.com/viewarticle/875216

20 www.bbc.co.uk/news/health-41011589

21 www.bbc.co.uk/news/health-41011589

22 www.telegraph.co.uk/health-fitness/body/vaginal-seeding-could-this-new-birth-trend-be-putting-babies-at/

23 Such as: onlinelibrary.wiley.com/doi/10.1111/j.1651-2227.2009.01371.x/full

24 clinicalepigeneticsjournal.biomedcentral.com/articles/10.1186/1868-7083-4-8

25 www.ncbi.nlm.nih.gov/pmc/articles/PMC1236800/#pmed-0020305-b1

26 www.ncbi.nlm.nih.gov/pubmed/9241315

27 There is some evidence to suggest that midwife-led antenatal care can improve outcomes for women: www.rcm.org.uk/news-views-and-analysis/news/vbac-more-likely-with-midwife-led-antenatal-care

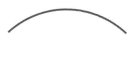

Index

Series editor: Susan Last

pinterandmartin.com